# THE
# CHRONIC
# COUGH
## ENIGMA

Also by Dr. Jamie Koufman

*Dropping Acid: The Reflux Diet Cookbook & Cure*

*Dr. Koufman's Acid Reflux Diet*

*Acid Reflux in Children*

# THE
# CHRONIC
# COUGH
## ENIGMA

Acid Reflux, Asthma, and Recalcitrant Cough
**THE PATH TO A CURE**

## DR. JAMIE KOUFMAN

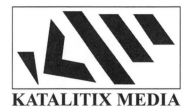

**KATALITIX MEDIA**

Copyright © 2014, 2021 Katalitix Media

ISBN 978-1-940561-00-4

ebook ISBN 978-1-940561-01-1

Published by Katalitix Media

Printed in the United States of America

Distributed by Simon & Schuster

NOTICE AND DISCLAIMER

This book is intended as a reference volume, not as a medical manual. The information is designed to help you make informed decisions about your health. It is not intended as a substitute for any diagnostics or treatments prescribed by your doctor. If you suspect that you have a medical problem, we urge you to seek medical help. Any use of this book is at the reader's discretion, as the advice and strategies contained within may not be suitable for every individual.

Mention of specific companies, products, organizations, or authorities in this book does not imply endorsement by the author or the publisher, nor does mention of specific companies, organizations, or authorities imply that they endorse this book.

Third Printing March 2021

For additional information, see: www.JamieKoufman.com and www.KoufmanConsulting.com

Dedicated to all the patients who have
taught me about chronic cough

# CONTENTS

# FOREWORD

The foreword of a book comes first and tells the reader what lies ahead. For me to be able to write this particular foreword seems perfect, and I will tell you why. I am sixty-two years old, but until two years ago I was afraid to look *forward*. I was afraid to try anything that might bring on an asthma attack.

For as long as I can remember, I had suffered from what many doctors told me was asthma. I never left the house without my inhaler and pills, my rescue kit in case an attack came on. If I laughed too hard I would start wheezing. If I went snorkeling I would start wheezing. As I got older it seemed anything and everything I did would bring on an asthma attack.

Now as you know, my professional life is spent in front of live audiences. As time went on I could barely get through a talk or TV show without gasping for breath. If you watch my PBS special *The Money Class* closely, you will hear and see me gasping for breath between every sentence.

My life started to come to a close. For over one year I stopped taking speaking engagements. My shows took forever to complete. To say I was in trouble was putting it mildly.

And then my first glimmer of hope appeared—a doctor recommended to me by Dr. Oz told me that I might have reflux.

Are you kidding?

Just imagine my reaction to this after countless doctors had told me the opposite for years. Well, thank God I listened to him and my journey to find a great reflux doctor began. Unfortunately, one GI doctor after another examined me and recommended the same little "purple pill," which didn't help at all.

Feeling totally lost, I found a book by Dr. Jamie Koufman called *Dropping Acid: The Reflux Diet Cookbook & Cure.* I read the book and with every page I turned, I thought, "*Wow*, this doctor makes total sense. I need to go see her."

So now let's jump ahead two years.

Dr. Jamie saved my life. This may sound dramatic but it is exactly how I feel. When you are gasping for breath, unable to speak, sleep, or do much, your life takes on a whole different meaning. And all of that changed for me, thanks to Dr. Jamie.

Treating reflux is complicated because there is far more to it than just popping a pill. What you eat, how you eat, and which (if any) medication is right for you is a science and Dr. Jamie is the rare expert.

So for those of you who have suffered from "asthma" for years, or those of you who already know you have reflux, there are real solutions that will allow you to live a life that you can look forward to each and every day.

Dr. Jamie, I thank you again and again for this book and for your insight into this devastating but curable disease.

Suze Orman

# PREFACE:
## WHY DOESN'T MY DOCTOR KNOW ABOUT THIS?

I f you have chronic cough and you have *not* already seen your doctor and had a chest x-ray, this book is *not* for you. And if you are a smoker with chronic cough, this book is probably *not* for you either.

I am not a lung doctor and this book is *not* about lung disease or asthma, but if in addition to cough, you have unexplained breathing problems or your "asthma" has not responded to treatment, then read on. This book is for people who have breathing problems and who have been coughing for months or years and cannot get useful answers.

• • •

When I first wrote *The Chronic Cough Enigma*, I had no idea it would be the only information of its kind available anywhere years later. It is an important book for several reasons. First, it gives chronic cough sufferers hope and a roadmap towards health. Second, it can be used to educate physicians. And third, it suggests that the future of healthcare needs to be re-consolidated, with the primary care physician (PCP) being put in charge of most common aerodigestive diseases. However, PCPs must be trained in *integrated aerodigestive medicine* (which I practice) so that expensive and ineffective specialists can be left out.

Chronic cough remains enigmatic because the medical community remains unaware that LPR (laryngopharyngeal reflux— today called *respiratory reflux*—is a major cause of chronic cough.

In addition, neurogenic cough also appears to remain invisible. It's rather like a medical black hole. And while there are only minor revisions in the text of this edition, my experience treating thousands of chronic cough patients has borne out all the observations and conclusions in this book.

Chronic cough—cough for more than four weeks—is an extremely common condition, but virtually the entire medical establishment remains clueless how to diagnose and manage *non-pulmonary cough*. Non-pulmonary? Most people with chronic cough are non-smokers with no lung disease, and that is the definition of "non-pulmonary." And by the way, non-pulmonary cough is more common than the pulmonary type.

Over the last few years, I have received hundreds of letters from strangers thanking me for the book that helped them get well. In addition, many chronic coughers buy copies of *The Chronic Cough Enigma* for their physicians. They educate their doctors to be able to help them. And yes, I have had thank you notes from physicians, too.

So, one might ask who is the audience for this book? And the answer now appears to be doctors and patients. This book, and specifically clinical use of the diagnostic indices (pages 12–14), especially the *Koufman Chronic Cough Index* could be used by all physicians involved in treating cough, including pulmonologists (lung doctors), otolaryngologists (ear, nose, and throat doctors), allergists, pediatricians, critical care specialists, and "generalists." i.e. PCPs and family physicians.

Just saying the word "cough," you'd think that the go-to physician would still be the pulmonologist, but lung doctors seem to know nothing about reflux-related and neurogenic cough. It's just not in their curriculum.

How could it be that medical specialists who deal with the airway know so little about it? The problem, at least in the United

States, is over-specialization. Indeed, when it comes to respiratory reflux and chronic cough, the specialist model of American medicine has failed. That's because the idea of dividing the body up into small, non-overlapping, anatomic areas makes no sense. The respiratory and digestive systems are intimately connected, and specialists don't seem to know that.

The evolution of my personal medical practice as an expert in acid reflux that affects the throat and airway, i.e. LPR, silent reflux, respiratory reflux (all terms that I coined) helped me see that silent, usually nighttime, respiratory reflux was ubiquitous and that it was the single most common cause of chronic cough. It is also the single most common cause of "allergies," "asthma," "sinus disease," and true sleep apnea.

• • •

The development of new medical technology and medical specialization occurred in parallel and in giant leaps since the 1970s. It's not clear which was the chicken and which was the egg, that is, which catalyzed which. In 1975, however, the Olympus Company made available for the first time quality endoscopes that allowed gastrointestinal specialists (GIs, gastroenterologists) to perform colonoscopies and upper gastrointestinal examinations (EGD, esophagogastroduodenoscopy).

With anatomic compartmentalization by specialist societies, the gastroenterologist became the physician for reflux. Indeed, they more-or-less took reflux over, and the GI mantra became, "Reflux is heartburn, heartburn is reflux, it's esophageal, and we own it." By the way, today, GI endoscopy is a multi-billion-dollar industry. Why is there no overlap between the specialties? Because physicians divided up the body so as to avoid competition and turf battles.

When I started publishing my work on LPR, including the

*magnum opus* of my career, *The Otolaryngologic Manifestations of GERD* (1991), in which I introduced throat acid pH-monitoring and provided patient data, GI naysayers began to flourish. (In those days, I still called LPR "GERD.") And for many years opinion leaders in GI rejected the notion that reflux could affect the airway, perhaps because that might threaten the GI reflux model.

*The problem is that only 17% of patients with reflux have heartburn and indigestion, which means more than four out of five reflux patients have LPR and not GERD.* Because GIs have no accurate test for LPR, all the other airway specialists are handicapped in its diagnosis. After all, if the pulmonologist suspects reflux, she/he is going to send the patient to a GI who unfortunately has nothing to offer the "respiratory reflux" patient.

• • •

It is important to note that although respiratory reflux is the most common cause of chronic cough, there are other causes, with the second most common being *neurogenic cough*. Because I am a laryngologist (voice/throat doctor) I became aware that partial paralysis of the vocal cords, so-called paresis, was common and often associated with a preceding viral infection at or near the onset of the chronic cough.

Here's the explanation in a nutshell: Anatomically, there are twelve *cranial nerves*. These nerves come out of the brain and account for all our senses as well as other functions. The 10th cranial nerve is called the *vagus nerve* and it is a powerhouse among nerves. That's because the vagus controls all the respiratory and digestive tracts (with the exception of the diaphragm). And the vagus nerves live just under the lining membranes of the throat so that they are vulnerable to damage from upper respiratory infections (viruses) and other causes.

When the patient has a history of an upper respiratory infection preceding onset of chronic cough, I will usually find vocal paresis and evidence that the vagus nerves have been infected or damaged. But again, the problem is there is no doctor for the vagus nerve. It basically involves all specialties that deal with the respiratory and digestive systems . . . again, specialists too specialized. However, I now have a lot of experience managing neurogenic cough, which is a type of "sick nerve syndrome." By the way, neurologists (nerve doctors) are equally uninformed about the vagus. The *Koufman Chronic Cough Index* is especially helpful to diagnose people with neurogenic cough, who may or may not have reflux, too. It is worth noting that in general, wet (productive) cough is usually reflux, and dry cough is usually neurogenic. Neurogenic cough is curable as is reflux, but the treatments are different.

• • •

Finally, although this book is about non-pulmonary chronic cough, respiratory reflux can cause or complicate lung disease, and it is often its root cause. Respiratory reflux is a major cause of all airway diseases. For example, the majority of patients with real asthma have reflux that may be an actual trigger of the asthma attacks. In addition, respiratory reflux can cause chronic bronchitis, emphysema, and even lung cancer. I refer the reader to my blog, www.JamieKoufman.com, for more information about the protean pulmonary manifestations of respiratory reflux, and to consult Dr. Koufman, go to www.KoufmanConsulting.com.

Jamie Koufman, M.D., F.A.C.S

# INTRODUCTION
## ARE YOU AN ENIGMA?

e·nig·ma *n.*
> 1: a puzzling or inexplicable occurrence or situation
> 2: a person of puzzling, incongruous, or inexplicable nature

Afraid to go to a movie or concert because your loud and disruptive cough will embarrass you? Do people turn away from you in elevators and other public places because they're afraid they will catch some awful disease? Have your trips to doctors, specialist after specialist, yielded nothing? If you or a loved one has been coughing for months or years and can't get medical help, this book is for you.

*Chronic cough* is one of the most common reasons for a person to seek medical attention and it can be disabling. Unfortunately, today millions of people with chronic cough remain misdiagnosed and untreated. The reasons for this are fragmentation of medicine due to overspecialization and a general failure of physicians to recognize, diagnose, and treat *neurogenic cough* (chapter 4) and *reflux-related cough* (chapter 5).

While there are doctors who specialize in diseases of the chest and lungs (*pulmonologists*), chronic cough is often *non-pulmonary*; that is, lung disease is not the root cause of the cough. Indeed, once a pulmonologist declares a patient's chronic cough to be non-pulmonary, there is no doctor for that patient.

**Chronic cough is enigmatic for most doctors, and by the time these patients get to me, they are usually frustrated, fearful, and angry.**

Most of my cough patients have seen a dozen or more specialists and have endured many worthless and expensive diagnostic tests and futile treatments. Unfortunately, most physicians are unable to diagnose silent airway reflux or neurogenic cough (caused by *vagal nerve* problems), the most common causes of chronic cough.

Despite the fact that I was trained as an *otolaryngologist,* an *ENT (ear, nose, and throat) physician,* the chief complaint of 20 percent of my patients is chronic cough. I am a chronic cough expert because I have evolved as an outlier physician. I am a *laryngologist* (voice and throat specialist) with decades of experience managing the toughest and seemingly incurable silent reflux and chronic cough patients in America.

**The ideas and approach presented in this book have already been rejected by the medical mainstream.**

Indeed, I was motivated to write this book because I was unable to get my research paper "The Diagnosis and Management of Non-Pulmonary Chronic Cough"[1] published. In it, I reported that 40 percent of the patients I saw had reflux-related cough; 14 percent had neurogenic cough; and 46 percent had both.[1]

The paper was rejected outright. One reviewer suggested that I simply must have missed pulmonary pathology, and another suggested that chronic cough was a psychological problem, a habituated neurotic behavior.

The peer-review process in this case may have broken down because I was expressing revolutionary ideas. I was asking my otolaryngologist colleagues to take responsibility for non-pulmonary chronic cough patients. In rejecting the paper, the journal's editor wrote: "The focus of this paper is too broad for our journal." In other words, the journal appeared to be simply begging off the chronic cough question.

This is not the first book I have written for patients that bypassed the medical establishment. My book *Dropping Acid: The*

*Reflux Diet Cookbook & Cure*[2] has overturned many of the accepted premises about *acid reflux*. Most doctors, for example, think that reflux is an incurable, chronic disease for which the only treatment is lifelong medication. Not true. Reflux is curable with healthy diet and lifestyle[3]; and by the way, it is the single most common cause of chronic cough.[1] More about that later.

The most frequent question my patients ask is "Why didn't my doctor know about this?" which is another reason I wrote this book.

**My goal is to empower frustrated patients to self-diagnose, but even after the diagnosis, it may be difficult to get appropriate treatment.**

And if, along the way, you discover that your *asthma* isn't really asthma, you're in good company. As you will see in chapter 7, "asthma" is one of the most common misdiagnoses in America— it's usually silent airway reflux!

This book is an extension of the original, unpublished chronic cough manuscript, written for chronic cough sufferers. The original paper presented the histories, findings, diagnostic testing results, and treatments of fifty consecutive chronic cough patients.[1] Those fifty effectively represent my experience with thousands of such patients and so this book integrates my entire professional experience as a clinician and researcher.[1–70]

I believe this book will provide a new and valuable window into the enigmatic chronic cough. I hope it is helpful to you, to someone you love, and to your physician. With accurate diagnosis, most chronic cough patients can be cured.

# THE
# CHRONIC
# COUGH
## ENIGMA

# I

# NON-PULMONARY
# CHRONIC COUGH

C hronic cough is one of the most common symptoms for which a patient seeks medical attention,[71] and yet a large proportion of such patients fail to receive an accurate diagnosis and effective treatment.[1, 71-76] Even pulmonologists (lung and chest specialists) and other medical specialists who deal with the airway, such as *allergists* and otolaryngologists, find chronic cough enigmatic.[72-76]

There are serious *pulmonary* causes of chronic cough such as *tuberculosis*, pneumonia, and lung cancer. So, if you have chronic cough and you haven't already seen your physician and had a chest X-ray, you must do so. You should also have a *TB* skin test.

**The first step in the diagnosis of chronic cough is to rule out a pulmonary cause. In this book non-pulmonary means that primary lung disease was already ruled out.**

*Recalcitrant* (refractory, hard to deal with) non-pulmonary chronic cough patients represent a significant proportion of my practice, and my list of the causes of non-pulmonary chronic cough is summarized in order of prevalence in table 1. In addition, these diagnoses are briefly discussed in Appendix B: What Else Could It Be?

The majority of cough patients referred to me by physicians are sent to rule in or rule out *silent airway reflux*, also known as *laryngopharyngeal reflux* (LPR). *Silent reflux* is the single most common cause of difficult-to-diagnose chronic cough, and neurogenic cough is the second most common cause. Diagnoses 3 through 7 in table 1 are relatively uncommon and diagnoses 8 through 13 are rare.

Remember, these are non-pulmonary causes of chronic cough. This bears repeating because pulmonary causes sometimes need to

## TABLE 1
# Causes of Non-Pulmonary Chronic Cough*

1. Airway Reflux, aka laryngopharyngeal reflux (LPR)

2. Neurogenic cough (2° post-viral vagal neuropathy)

3. Angiotensin converting enzyme (ACE) inhibitors

4. Aspiration due to glottal insufficiency (paralysis)

5. Asthma / Allergy / Sinusitis / Post-nasal drip

6. Zenker's or distal esophageal diverticulum

7. Occult bronchial foreign body

8. Tracheoesophageal fistula

9. Trachebronchial (e.g., carcinoid) tumor

10. Esophageal achalasia

11. Ortner's syndrome

12. Cerumen impaction

13. Syngamus laryngeus

*DISCLOSURE AND DISCLAIMER: This table represents a summary of the author's experience and is not intended to represent a complete list of all the possible causes and diagnoses of cough. Furthermore, it is acknowledged that the foci of this book are reflux-related and neurogenic cough, not other (especially pulmonary) causes.

be ruled out more than once. For example, if a chronic-cough patient comes to me for evaluation and she or he hasn't had a pulmonary evaluation for several years, at the very least I obtain a chest X-ray, TB skin test, and pulmonary function tests. I also commonly consult a pulmonologist.

Pulmonologists, however, don't know a lot about *non-pulmonary chronic cough.* The American College of Chest Physicians' *Management of Cough Clinical Practice Guidelines* concedes that the diagnosis and treatment of chronic cough remains challenging.[72]

> Not all diagnostic tests in predicting the cause of cough are known . . . sequential and additive therapy is often crucial because more than one cause of cough is frequently present. Marked improvement or resolution of cough is the *sine qua non* for success. Based upon this standard, it has been demonstrated that the use of empiric treatment, systematically directed at the common causes of cough works and is an important component of the successful approach to the diagnosis and treatment of cough.[72]

*Empiric treatment*—what is that? This means, for example, when antireflux medication is given to a patient believed to have reflux-related chronic cough, that medication will stop the reflux and hence stop the cough. Unfortunately, when it comes to chronic cough due to reflux into the airway (i.e., *LPR or "respiratory reflux"*), empiric antireflux treatment as a *therapeutic trial* simply doesn't work.[74, 75]

**Reflux treatment with *acid-suppressive medications* alone is not useful as a diagnostic test. If a chronic cougher does not respond to antireflux medication, it does not prove anything. Reflux may still be the cause of the cough.**

When it comes to reflux-related cough, the acidity (pH) of the *refluxate* is relatively unimportant as reflux into the airway at any level of acidity (or non-acidity) can trigger cough. *Aspiration* of even a small amount of a neutral-pH refluxate causes cough.

Another major source of confusion about the role and diagnosis of reflux in chronic cough stems from the fact that the *reflux-testing* methods in current use by *gastroenterologists* (GIs) and otolaryngologists (ENTs) are inaccurate. By examining my pH-monitoring data, I determined that the predictive value of any esophageal reflux test (alone) for airway reflux was only 49 percent.[67, 69] GI reflux-testing techniques lack *pharyngeal* (throat) reflux data and that is why esophageal pH monitoring is virtually useless.[67] Would you take or trust the results of a test that got it right less than half of the time?

## Airway Reflux Testing

In the reflux world, one of the biggest problems remaining is that most doctors are unable to diagnose airway reflux using clinical measures *and* they have no definitive diagnostic test for it. The diagnosis of airway reflux remains a huge black hole. And let me reiterate, esophageal (GI) tests for reflux just won't do!

In addition to using the symptoms and laryngeal findings (see below) to definitively diagnose airway reflux, one must detect *acid* and/or *pepsin* (the main stomach enzyme) in the throat.[2-4, 7, 28, 46, 49, 54, 58, 59, 61, 70] I test for both.

In my reflux-testing laboratory, I employ two new (designed specifically to detect airway reflux) reflux testing technologies. They are *high-definition airway and esophageal ISFET pH monitoring*, and a spit-in-a-cup pepsin assay.[70] The latter test, similar in concept and design to a pregnancy test, detects the stomach enzyme *pepsin*.[70] This assay, still in the final stages of development, is an ultra-sensitive test for airway reflux.[4, 70] Depending upon regulatory hurdles, this excellent diagnostic will hopefully become widely available soon.

The gold standard for diagnosing airway reflux, and determining its severity and pattern, is *ambulatory pH monitoring*.[5–7, 25, 45, 67] Before this test, I always perform high-definition *pharyngeal/UES/esophageal manometry*, which evaluates esophageal function, including valve function and coordination of the swallowing system. Manometry provides essential information, which often alters treatment.[25, 27] In many of my patients, poor esophageal valve function or poor esophageal function (*dysmotility*) requires specific treatment to get the system back in working order.[25, 27] Manometry also reveals precisely where to place the pH sensors for pH monitoring.

**Accurate pH data from the pharynx (throat) is essential for the diagnosis of airway reflux.**

Properly analyzed pH data is essential, and I use the best (*ISFET*) sensors for our pH monitoring.

The pH data from the unpublished chronic cough manuscript[1] showed that without pharyngeal data, I would have inaccurately concluded that most of the patients studied did not have reflux at all. Indeed, had I used GI reflux-testing criteria, that is, examined only esophageal pH data, two-thirds of the pH studies would have been incorrectly interpreted as normal.[1]

In reality, 86 percent of the group had pH-documented airway reflux.[1] And using pH<5 as the threshold (the traditional value is pH <4) for pharyngeal (throat) reflux, the reflux-related cough patients studied averaged over one hundred pharyngeal reflux episodes in the twenty-four-hour pH test. Now, that is indisputable proof of airway reflux in the chronic cough study group.[1] (I wish this airway reflux testing method was widely available, but not yet.)

## Clinical Diagnosis of Airway Reflux

A clinician experienced in managing silent airway reflux may find the symptoms and throat examination adequate to make a diagnosis.[7, 22, 23, 31, 39] Examination of the throat, specifically the *larynx* (voice box), will (when present) reveal findings of reflux, but most otolaryngologists (ENTs) do not appreciate those findings. I have been lecturing on this topic for years, and recently I tested my colleagues by showing an example of *reflux laryngitis* (figure 1A).

I asked the assembled ENT doctors, "Is this larynx (fig. 1A) abnormal or normal?" Almost no one responded. "Dear colleagues, either this larynx is normal or abnormal. Please put up your hand if you think it is abnormal." Again few hands went up. "Okay then, how many of you think that this larynx is normal?" Several hands were raised. After this no-response set of responses, I put up the photo of the normal larynx (fig. 1B) and announced that it was the same patient after successful reflux treatment.

The fact is that 95 percent of my ENT colleagues don't know what reflux in the throat looks like. Possibly they don't know what normal looks like—neither do gastroenterologists nor pulmonologists—because reflux is so ubiquitous.

As surprising as it may seem, this generally isn't taught in *otolaryngology* residency programs. So throat doctors don't yet appreciate the appearance of airway reflux. In fact, having shown this slide (fig. 1) at a number of national and international meetings to an estimated two thousand ENT doctors, I can say with certainty that very few otolaryngologists appreciate the findings of airway reflux.

**Figure 1: Laryngeal Findings of Reflux and Normal.**
**Before and After Treatment (Same Patient)**

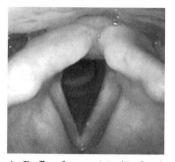 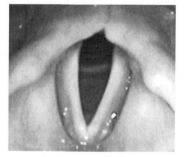

| A. Reflux laryngitis (Before) | B. Normal (After) |

*These before- and after-treatment photographs show the larynx of a woman with airway reflux who presented with chronic cough and "asthma." The V-like structures are the vocal cords. A: The pre-treatment vocal cords are swollen with a sausagelike appearance. B: By comparison the photo on the right (after reflux treatment) shows the normal thin appearance of the vocal cords, shaped rather like the bow of a ship. (see also: www.JamieKoufman.com)*

**This failure of most ENT doctors to recognize the findings of airway reflux remains a serious problem for patients with chronic cough.**

It is even worse for gastroenterologists. GIs don't examine the throat at all and they have no test for airway reflux. In fact, GIs know almost nothing about airway reflux, and some even have difficulty believing it. In addition, GIs still think that diagnostic tests for esophageal reflux can be applied to patients with reflux-related cough; that is, airway reflux. But esophageal tests for airway reflux are useless.

To return to the question of empiric treatment as a therapeutic trial, its failure as a diagnostic maneuver is also because acid-suppression (increasing the pH of the refluxed material) does not stop airway reflux from occurring, and essential *lifestyle factors* (such as night eating) are not corrected by the use of *antireflux medication* alone.[1, 67]

To date, because there is no generally available and reliable diagnostic for airway reflux, the medical and scientific literature (in pulmonology, otolaryngology, and gastroenterology) has not conclusively addressed the causal relationship between airway reflux and chronic cough.[1, 72–77] To my knowledge, the only place where specific and accurate airway reflux testing is being performed today is in my office.

Before moving on to discuss the diagnosis of chronic cough, it is important to mention that there are significant relationships between airway reflux, *upper respiratory infections* (URIs), *vagal nerve dysfunction*, and cough.[18, 78]

**Viral inflammation of the "cough (vagus) nerve" and airway reflux, individually or together, can cause chronic cough. These connections will be highlighted in Chapter 3: Post-Viral Vagal Neuropathy.**

In summary, the specialty-fragmented healthcare system does not understand the non-pulmonary chronic cough patient, and the physicians who should be the go-to doctors for such patients—pulmonologists, allergists, otolaryngologists, gastroenterologists—are not attuned to the diagnosis and treatment of reflux-related and neurogenic cough. Furthermore, most physicians, regardless of their medical specialty, have no diagnostic tests for such neurogenic problems or for airway reflux.

# 2
# DIAGNOSIS AND THE
# CHRONIC COUGH INDEX

What do I do first when I see a new patient with chronic cough? For the past thirty-five years, I have been asking new patients to fill out quick, customized, nononsense questionnaires. The first of these questionnaires was the *reflux symptom index* (RSI),[39] designed to identify airway reflux (laryngopharyngeal reflux, LPR), particularly silent airway reflux. The RSI is a validated *outcomes instrument*,[39] and I have asked my patients to fill it out at every visit for as long as I can remember because the RSI is an excellent measure of airway reflux symptoms.

Here is an example:

A thirty-three-year-old male psychologist came to see me with symptoms of *globus* (a sensation of a lump in the throat), *choking episodes*, and chronic cough. His RSI was 35 (greater than 15 is abnormal) and his throat examination showed severe reflux. This patient typically ate dinner very late because of his work. I placed him on a strict detox reflux diet (see Chapter 6: Dr. Koufman's Reflux Boot Camp), which includes no eating and no lying down within four hours of bed. Three weeks later, he was feeling great and his RSI was down to 5. From 35 to 5 in a few weeks is a very good treatment result!

I always use the RSI to help track my reflux patients' progress. The first thing that I check at every visit is whether the RSI is better, worse, or the same. Since its publication in 2002, the RSI has become one of the most widely used symptom indices for airway reflux in the world.

Since I also take care of many patients with voice disorders, I came up with a comparable diagnostic index for *glottal insuffiency* (symptoms caused when the vocal cords do not close properly).

This index, the *glottal closure index* (GCI),[55] is an especially sensitive measure of symptoms caused by *vocal cord paralysis* or *paresis* (weakness, partial paralysis), common in people with voice disorders. The diagnoses of reflux and/or vocal cord paresis account for the majority of patients with both *voice disorders* and chronic cough.

A sixty-six-year-old clergyman came to see me with a left vocal cord paralysis caused by thyroid cancer surgery. The surgeon had to remove the vocal cord nerve to get the tumor out. The patient spoke with a barely audible whisper; his GCI was 20, with greater than 8 being abnormal. In addition, he was having trouble with aspiration (food going down the wrong pipe.) A few days later, I operated on this patient, performing a vocal cord repositioning procedure to restore his voice.[79, 80] When he came back the following week to have his stitches removed, he was very happy to have his old voice back, and his GCI was down to 3. Indeed, the GCI is a good measure of vocal cord function.

A few years ago, I realized that my practice included a large number of patients with chronic cough, and that I was asking every chronic cough patient questions designed to differentiate reflux-related from neurogenic cough.[1]

For example, do you awaken from a sound sleep coughing violently and gasping for air like a fish out of water? This is caused by airway reflux and only airway reflux. It is not asthma (see Chapter 7: Asthma That Isn't Asthma). Coughing after eating, when lying down, or bending over is also typical of reflux-related cough.

On the other hand, do you cough when entering an air-conditioned room or when chuckling or talking? This is typical of neurogenic cough. Continual daytime coughing, or coughing when exposed to certain fumes such as perfume or automobile exhaust is also characteristic of neurogenic cough.

Remember the fifty patients systematically studied in the original chronic cough paper?[1] Well, 14 percent had neurogenic cough (alone), 40 percent had reflux-related cough (alone), and 46 percent had both neurogenic and reflux-related cough.[1] (Be patient and read on; those diagnoses are covered in chapters 4 and 5.)

Before coming to see me, most chronic cough patients have never even heard the words *neurogenic cough*. And airway reflux is usually overlooked as a cause of cough. In fact, most reflux-related-cough patients have been mistakenly told that they didn't have reflux by a gastroenterologist who applied GI (esophageal, GERD) diagnostic criteria to an airway reflux patient. The focus of this book is on reflux-related and neurogenic cough because these are the main causes of non-pulmonary chronic cough.

**All my chronic cough patients fill out the glottal closure index, the reflux symptom index, and the *chronic cough index* forms, and you should too. Take all three quizzes now.**

These indices should provide you with a presumptive diagnosis or diagnoses. And the chapters that follow should help you unravel the mystery, the enigma, of your cough.

Please, circle one answer for each and every question. Don't leave any questions out; answer them all; no little arrows or maybes.

## TABLE 2

# The Glottal Closure Index (GCI)

**How do the following affect you? 0 = No Problem  5 = Severe Problem**

| | | | | | | |
|---|---|---|---|---|---|---|
| Speaking takes extra effort | 0 | 1 | 2 | 3 | 4 | 5 |
| Throat discomfort or pain after using your voice | 0 | 1 | 2 | 3 | 4 | 5 |
| Vocal fatigue, voice weakens as you talk | 0 | 1 | 2 | 3 | 4 | 5 |
| Voice cracks or sounds different | 0 | 1 | 2 | 3 | 4 | 5 |

**Circle one number on each of the four lines above.**
**Now, add up your four numbers to get your GCI:** _____

If your GCI is 8 or greater, you are likely to have vocal cords that are not closing properly from aging, atrophy, scarring, paresis, paralysis, or because of a vocal cord growth of some kind.

## TABLE 3
# The Reflux Symptom Index (RSI)

**How do the following affect you? 0 = No Problem  5 = Severe Problem**

| | | | | | | |
|---|---|---|---|---|---|---|
| Hoarseness or a problem with your voice | 0 | 1 | 2 | 3 | 4 | 5 |
| Clearing your throat | 0 | 1 | 2 | 3 | 4 | 5 |
| Excess throat mucous or postnasal drip | 0 | 1 | 2 | 3 | 4 | 5 |
| Difficulty swallowing food, liquids, pills | 0 | 1 | 2 | 3 | 4 | 5 |
| Coughing after you eat or after lying down | 0 | 1 | 2 | 3 | 4 | 5 |
| Breathing difficulty or choking episodes | 0 | 1 | 2 | 3 | 4 | 5 |
| Troublesome or annoying cough | 0 | 1 | 2 | 3 | 4 | 5 |
| Sensation of a lump in your throat | 0 | 1 | 2 | 3 | 4 | 5 |
| Heartburn, chest pain, or indigestion | 0 | 1 | 2 | 3 | 4 | 5 |

**Circle one number on each of the lines above.**
**Now, add up your numbers to get your RSI:** _____

If you have an RSI score of 15 or greater, you have a 90 percent chance of having reflux by specialized reflux testing.

## TABLE 4

# Voice Institute of New York
# Chronic Cough Index

**Please circle Yes or No for all ten questions (no maybes). Add up the answers in each column to derive the REFLUX-to-NEUROGENIC ratio.**

| | | |
|---|---|---|
| Do you awaken from a sound sleep coughing violently, with or without trouble breathing? | Yes | No |
| Do you have choking episodes when you cannot get enough air, gasping for air? | Yes | No |
| Do you usually cough when you lie down in bed, or when you just lie down to rest? | Yes | No |
| Do you usually cough after meals or eating? | Yes | No |
| Do you cough when (or after) you bend over? | Yes | No |
| Do you more or less cough all day long? | No | Yes |
| Does change of temperature make you cough? | No | Yes |
| Does laughing or chuckling cause you to cough? | No | Yes |
| Do fumes (perfume, automobile fumes, burned toast, etc.) cause you to cough? | No | Yes |
| Does speaking, singing, or talking on the phone cause you to cough? | No | Yes |
| **Add the circles in each column (there must be 10 circles) to determine your Reflux-to-Neurogenic (R : N) Ratio** | R | N |
| R_____ : _____N | | |

If we examine the three indices (GCI, RSI, CCI), a pattern will emerge. First, look at your answers to the GCI. If your GCI score is 8 or more, you probably have a voice problem. When is your voice better and when is it worse? Morning *hoarseness* is typical for people who reflux during the night. Vocal fatigue and hoarseness that gets worse as the day goes on is more typical of *vocal cord paresis* (weakness) and *post-viral vagal neuropathy* (PVVN). If you have PVVN, you are likely to have a *neurogenic* component to your cough. (PVVN is important and is the topic of the next chapter.)

Second, examine your RSI. Now that you know the symptoms of silent airway reflux, do you have it? You may never have *heartburn* or *indigestion*, but you still may have a reflux-related cough. Generally, if you have an RSI score of 15 or greater, there is a 90 percent chance you have reflux.[67]

Finally, examine your CCI, add up the two columns and find your reflux-to-neurogenic (R:N) ratio. The two numbers should always add up to 10.

**If your R:N ratio is 10:0 (or even 9:1 or 8:2), you most certainly have reflux as the primary cause of your cough. Conversely, if your R:N ratio is 0:10 (or even 1:9 or 2:8), you most certainly have a neurogenic cough. All other scores imply that you probably have both reflux-related and neurogenic cough.**

You will see in the chapters that follow, that neurogenic does not mean psychogenic (a psychological cause). Neurogenic simply means "of or relating to a nerve," and in the case of neurogenic cough, it is the vagus nerve that is out of whack.

If your R:N ratio ranges from 7:3 to 3:7 (i.e., 7:3, 6:4, 5:5, 4:6, 3:7), you probably have both reflux-related and neurogenic cough. Amazing as it may seem, the CCI gives the correct diagnosis most of the time.

Now that you have a possible diagnosis, the next chapter on

post-viral vagal neuropathy (PVVN) will help explain how and why neurogenic and reflux-related cough begin following an upper respiratory infection (URI).

Understanding how the *aerodigestive* system is affected by vagus nerve problems is key to understanding chronic cough.

**One big difference between reflux-related and neurogenic cough is that neurogenic cough is almost always dry, whereas refluxers often have some degree of chronic bronchitis and therefore a wet cough. Yes, airway refluxers do actually reflux into their lungs.**

Reflux itself can cause lung problems such as chronic bronchitis, pneumonia (COPD), and idiopathic pulmonary fibrosis. After all, if you are refluxing into your throat and airway, particularly during sleep, the refluxate is getting into your lungs as well.

Remember, if you haven't had a chest X-ray and a TB skin test, see your doctor and get them done.

**It is interesting that so many elderly people in nursing homes die of "community-acquired pneumonia." Community-acquired implies that no pathologic organism (bacteria) was identified. Here's what I think: give an elderly refluxer a bedtime snack, chocolate pudding and ginger ale, for instance, and that's what ends up in their lungs at two o'clock in the morning—it's chocolate-pudding–ginger-ale pneumonia.**

If you are a smoker, the above indices may be less accurate because smoking (alone) is a common cause of chronic bronchitis and cough. In other words, chronic cough in smokers is usually due to a primary pulmonary (lung) cause of the cough and this book is about non-pulmonary chronic cough.

# 3
# POST-VIRAL VAGAL
# NEUROPATHY

This chapter is about a common problem, post-viral vagal neuropathy (PVVN); I coined the term in 1991.[18] Like silent reflux, this condition remains relatively underdiagnosed. What is PVVN?

**Common upper respiratory infections caused by viruses can damage nerves in the throat (namely the vagus nerves) that control all respiratory and digestive functions, including speaking, singing, swallowing, reflux, asthma, and cough.**

Here is a case example:

A twenty-five-year-old female grammar school teacher came to see me with a nine-month history of a sensation of a lump in her throat, breathy hoarseness (*dysphonia*), vocal fatigue, intense pain with voice use (*odynophonia*), and cough.

Her cough, voice, and odynophonia made it hard for her to get through the day. By the afternoon, she was miserable, and by the end of the week she was in tears because of her voice and throat pain.

Nine months earlier, she had been completely healthy with no symptoms whatsoever; her problems began following an upper respiratory infection (URI). She described having a cold that turned into severe laryngitis and *pleurisy*. Weeks later when she started teaching, she was already having severe symptoms that just grew worse as the school year wore on.

When she came to see me, she was desperate. From my initial patient intake forms, I saw that her reflux symptom index (RSI) of 33 was very high (normal <15), indicating severe reflux. Her glottal closure index (GCI) of 18 was also very high (normal <8), meaning that she had vocal cord problems too.

The GCI measures voice symptoms and is very useful in determining if a person has problems with the vocal cord nerves, specifically if the vocal cords are paralyzed or partly paralyzed. This patient's high GCI of 18 suggested that she likely had vagus nerve damage.

Examination of the voice box by *transnasal flexible laryngoscopy* (TFL) confirmed that she had a *paretic* (weak, partially paralyzed) left vocal cord. Special vocal cord function testing called *stroboscopy* showed that the left vocal cord was floppy, also indicating *vocal cord paresis*. Finally, her larynx showed severe reflux.

The patient underwent tests for reflux and for vocal cord paresis (e.g., *laryngeal electromyography*), all of which indicated that she had suffered a post-viral vagal neuropathy.

To complete this clinical anecdote, the patient responded well to an intense antireflux program and to two medications used to treat neurogenic cough and vagal neuropathies (*amitriptyline* 10 mg. before bed, and *gabapentin* 100 mg. four times a day). The drugs were given in this case for her cough and throat pain. Within six weeks, she was asymptomatic and within six months, she was off all medication.

## Laryngeal Electromyography (LEMG)

I have been performing *laryngeal electromyography* (LEMG) on a daily basis since 1987, and I believe that I have learned much of what I know about vagal nerve problems and PVVN[18] from LEMG.[17] For several years, I worked with a neurologist who specialized in electromyography to learn how to interpret the test.

LEMG is the only definitive test to determine the cause, severity, and prognosis of nerve problems, especially vagal dysfunction, i.e., PVVN.[17, 18] It is a slightly uncomfortable procedure during which fine needle electrodes are inserted into the laryngeal muscles through the skin of the neck. Fortunately, this area is not particularly sensitive and LEMG is performed quickly.

LEMG positively confirms the diagnosis of PVVN. For most patients, PVVN shows an old *polyneuropathy* involving most, often all, of the four laryngeal nerves. Old means that the nerve is unlikely to recover fully or to worsen; the nerve problem is stable. This pattern suggests that the underlying cause must have been a throat problem, such as a viral infection, in order to involve just those nerves in that way.

LEMG can also reveal any ongoing, unstable neurological process.[17] When the LEMG demonstrates a pattern of *spontaneous activity*, this suggests the possibility of a serious condition such as thyroid cancer, brain tumor, Lyme disease, or MS (multiple sclerosis). Tumors tend to affect just one nerve or just one side. Whenever I find spontaneous activity, I usually order special tests such as MRIs, CT scans, and sometimes referral to a *neurologist*.

One final benefit of LEMG is that it reveals the prognosis for recovery after a nerve injury has occurred.

Until now, I have been reluctant to report my LEMG results in my chronic cough patients, because almost all have evidence of PVVN. I suspect that vagal neuropathies are very common, affecting about half of the general population. This area needs more research, but unfortunately few clinicians perform LEMG.

LEMG is another important diagnostic test that has just fallen through the cracks. Neurologists seldom do LEMG because they don't know how to place the needle electrodes in the larynx, and most otolaryngologists don't want to learn LEMG either (perhaps because the reimbursement for LEMG is relatively low).

This chapter on post-viral vagal neuropathy may feel like a speed bump at this point in the book because PVVN is relatively complicated and can be difficult to understand. However, it is necessary to put vagal function and dysfunction in context or you will have trouble understanding the crucial role of the vagus in the development of symptoms such as neurogenic cough.

What is neurogenic, and how can we put PVVN in perspective? Have you ever seen *Bell's palsy*? It is a droopy paralysis of one side of the face caused by a viral infection. Some people report that they had a coldlike illness first and others do not. Nevertheless, Bell's palsy is caused by a viral infection of the facial nerve such that the nerve itself gets infected, swollen, and stops working.

PVVN may be thought of as Bell's palsy of the throat. The vagus nerves reside just under the lining membranes of the throat and may easily be infected by any virulent virus. This is how we think PVVN occurs and explains the LEMG pattern of a polyneuropathy.

Another point of comparison between PVVN and Bell's palsy is that some people with Bell's palsy do not make a full spontaneous recovery and are left with subtle or not so subtle facial asymmetry. The same is true of PVVN. Sometimes after the nerves heal, there are crossed wires, and those improperly directed nerves can lead to cough, pain, or other neurogenic symptoms.

**Besides cough, there are several other common vagal neurogenic symptoms, such as burning tongue, chronic sore (burning) throat, and painful speaking (odynophonia).**

Another interesting parallel between Bell's palsy and PVVN is that both may or may not be associated with a preceding upper respiratory infection (URI). About half of my PVVN patients have a clear history of a URI at the onset and about half don't. In the latter case, how then do I know the diagnosis of PVVN is correct?

The answer is that the clinical syndrome is similar with or

without the history of a prior viral illness. The key features of PVVN follow:

1. Relatively sudden onset of airway reflux with elevated RSI
2. Glottal closure (voice) symptoms with elevated GCI
3. Findings of reflux on laryngeal examination and other diagnostics, such as pH monitoring
4. Findings of vocal cord paresis (weakness) on laryngeal examination and laryngeal electromyography

Many of my chronic cough patients clearly date the onset of the cough to a preceding URI. In addition, there are many patients with acute-onset of airway reflux (without chronic cough) after having had a URI.

Almost all PVVN patients have moderately severe *glottal closure* symptoms (GCI of >10) and demonstrable vocal cord paresis (weakness) on both laryngeal examination and laryngeal electromyography.

While reflux alone can cause serious voice disturbances, more than half of my chronic cough patients have voice problems. After diagnostic testing, these are almost always in the PVVN group. Why is this important? Vocal cord paresis is a manifestation of nerve damage either to the branches of the nerve(s) going to the voice box or to the larger nerve, the vagus, itself.

The vagus nerve is the X[th] cranial nerve, and it may be adversely affected by a URI. The vagus is the "cough nerve," and it is amazingly complex; it is a *sensory, motor,* and *autonomic nerve.* (*Autonomic* essentially means "automatic"; for example, once initiated, swallowing is an automatic or autonomic function powered by the vagus.)

Much of my medical practice is devoted to diagnosing and

treating vagal nerve problems. Before I even meet and begin to assess a new chronic cough patient, I already have a lot of information from the reflux symptom index, the chronic cough index, and the glottal closure index they filled out before seeing me. The CCI index, with its reflux-to-neurogenic ratio, suggests a diagnosis or diagnoses, and the RSI and GCI help confirm the correct diagnoses and their possible causes.

The vagus runs the show. It is the reflux nerve; it's the vocal cord paresis nerve; it's the globus nerve; it's the swallowing problem nerve; it's the slow stomach (*gastroparesis*) nerve; it's the asthma nerve; it's the reactive airways nerve; and it is always the cough nerve.

The high prevalence of PVVN in my patients with chronic cough suggests that vagal nerve testing and airway reflux testing should be used in the evaluation of such patients. The era of blind empiric therapy for chronic cough that began generations ago should now give way to more precise diagnosis and customized treatment.

Even without a history of a prior viral infection, PVVN is still a discrete clinical syndrome that I recognize and diagnose using a battery of tests (e.g., *videostroboscopy*, laryngeal electromyography). It is not widely recognized by physicians, including neurologists (nerve doctors). I recommend that my PVVN patients do not see neurologists, because PVVN is an isolated problem and not part of an ongoing or systemic neurological disease process.

That said, there are some people who present with vagal nerve problems (not PVVN pattern) who do have serious medical diseases. Brain tumors, Lyme disease, thyroid and lung cancer, for example, can all affect the vagal nerves and can cause vocal cord paresis. Clinically, such serious conditions do not resemble PVVN.

In summary, people who have post-viral or relatively sudden-onset airway reflux symptoms revealed by the RSI and glottal closure (voice) symptoms by the GCI usually will have a clinical diagnosis of post-viral vagal neuropathy.

# 4

# NEUROGENIC COUGH

Neurogenic (nerve-caused) cough is rarely properly diagnosed and treated, and yet it is the sole cause of 14 percent of my chronic cough cases.[1] Neurogenic cough is a kind of "sick nerve syndrome," commonly associated with PVVN. Yes, vagal dysfunction is the root cause of neurogenic cough.

A forty-year-old business woman from England came to see me with a ten-year history of chronic cough. She had a severe cold at the onset of her cough. She coughed all day, every day, but did not cough at night. She reported that the cough was dry and a frequent tickling feeling in her throat triggered the coughing. Change of temperature, such as entering an air-conditioned room, and perfume also triggered her cough.

She had previously seen two internists, an allergist, two pulmonologists, four otolaryngologists, and three gastroenterologists. Among her misdiagnoses were allergies, asthma, reflux, and psychogenic cough. When she came to see me she was otherwise healthy and on no medications. Her glottal closure index was 8 (mildly abnormal) and her reflux symptom index was normal.

Examination of her larynx revealed mild bilateral (both-sided) vocal cord paresis and no findings of airway reflux. Laryngeal electromyography showed a polyneuropathy affecting all four laryngeal nerves. I asked her, "Have you ever heard the term neurogenic cough?" She had not.

I placed her on a small dose of amitriptyline (10 mg.) at bedtime and nothing else. In two days, this completely stopped her ten-year cough. I left her on medication for almost ten months and then discontinued it. Now, five years later, she remains free from coughing.

After ten years of coughing and so many doctors, how could this case be so easily solved? Why did the medicine work so quickly and why didn't her cough return when the medicine was discontinued?

Isolated neurogenic cough is almost always associated with vocal cord paresis and environmental triggers. In this case, the pattern of the cough and the finding of vocal cord paresis on laryngeal examination made me strongly suspect the diagnosis. The patient's almost unbelievably rapid and complete response to amitriptyline confirmed it.

While patients with neurogenic cough often get some benefit from amitriptyline, most need to have the dosage adjusted over time, and many need more than one medication. Amitriptyline is the cornerstone in the treatment of neurogenic cough and I often start at a dose of just 5 mg. But before discussing treatment in greater detail, I must first answer the question of why the cough did not return after cessation of the medication.

There is tremendous *neural plasticity* in the vagus nerve control center in the brain; it can change how it works over time. When a person has a neurogenic cough, the coughing sparks a cascade of nerve and brain responses like a string of firecrackers. The key to effectively curing neurogenic cough is to stop the cough and the neural cascade. If that can be done for three to nine months, the brain can reset, almost as if the thermostat was changed to a cooler, more comfortable temperature. While we do not fully understand how medicines like amitriptyline work, it is clear that they can reset chronic cough.

Again, in determining the correct diagnosis, the history and pattern of cough are most important. Certainly if the symptoms began after a URI, post-viral vagal neuropathy and a neurogenic cough is highly likely.

Here listed are the telltale red flags for neurogenic cough:

1. Cough from talking or singing
2. Cough caused by changes in temperature or air conditioning
3. Cough caused by perfume or other fumes
4. Presence of other neurogenic symptoms such as odynophonia (painful  speaking) or painful burning throat. (*Throatburn* is typically a neurogenic  symptom and not a common symptom of reflux.)

For the treatment of neurogenic cough, I generally use just three medications alone or in combination:

*Amitriptyline* (Elavil) is an old and still commonly prescribed medication in the class of drugs known as tricyclic antidepressants. Interestingly, today it is seldom used to treat depression and is usually prescribed for anxiety, tension, and migraine headaches. It is my first-choice drug for neurogenic cough.

*Gabapentin* (Neurontin). Although originally developed for treatment of epilepsy, gabapentin was never really prescribed for that purpose. Its primary use is for the treatment of *neurogenic* (*neuropathic*) *pain* such as neurogenic foot pain from diabetes and fibromyalgia. Fortunately, it appears to specifically improve vagal function and it is particularly effective for treating post-viral vagal neuropathic symptoms such as chronic sore throat, throatburn, burning tongue, odynophonia (painful speaking), and neurogenic cough. Gabapentin comes in a variety of doses that make it easily adjusted for each patient's needs.

I consider amitriptyline to be the cornerstone medication for treating neurogenic cough, even used in mini-doses (e.g., 2.5 to 5.0 mg., which is one-quarter to one-half of a 10 mg. pill). Small doses of amitriptyline seem to make other medications, particularly gabapentin—also given in small doses at bedtime—more effective.

For neurogenic cough, I almost always start with amitriptyline; although I do push the dose up in some cases, as long as the patient does not have side effects. It remains the single most effective one-drug treatment, and since it is usually given at bedtime, side effects (e.g., sleepiness, dry mouth) are uncommon. The mechanism of this drug's beneficial effect on neurogenic cough is unknown, but in these low doses, it is certainly not acting as an antidepressant.

When I talk to patients about starting treatment for neurogenic cough, I always explain that the recipe is different for everyone and the goal of treatment is to stop the cough completely. Treatment of neurogenic cough is somewhat like making soup; you never add too much salt, pepper, or sugar at the beginning, and the smallest effective dose of all medications is best. I never use any kind of narcotic analgesic such as codeine. or tramadol.

**If I am correct that PVVN is so common, many more people with chronic cough have reflux-related and neurogenic cough than neurogenic cough alone. Therefore, most of my reflux-related chronic cough patients are also treated for neurogenic cough. In fact, most people have both.**

Further, in my experience, allergies are not often a cause of chronic cough, but they do interact with neurogenic cough. The lining of the throat has receptors, like switches, that can trigger cough, and a host of different factors can influence the cough reflex. Allergies and even environmental factors such as air quality and particulates can set or reset the threshold for neurogenic cough.

Finally, although neurogenic cough can be worsened by stress, cough is almost never a psychological symptom. In my experience, there is no such thing as *psychogenic cough*.

# 5
# SILENT AIRWAY REFLUX

re·flux *n.* [L. *re-* back + *fluxus* flow]
    1: a flowing back
    2: process of refluxing

Acid reflux is the popular name for a condition that occurs as a result of the backflow of *gastric* (stomach) contents into the *esophagus* (the swallowing tube that connects the throat to the stomach) and the *airway* (breathing passages that include the nose, throat, vocal cords, bronchi, and lungs).

Reflux comes in many forms but the most important new discovery is that silent airway reflux affects almost one-in-five Americans.[3] People with silent airway reflux often have misdiagnosed symptoms and diseases. Do you have asthma that doesn't get better on asthma medication? Do you have sinus trouble and your surgery didn't help? Have you had misdiagnosed chronic cough that has defied effective treatment for years?

Silent Reflux is reflux that occurs without the obvious reflux symptoms of heartburn and indigestion. Most people are unaware that they have it, and most doctors never think of it as a cause of many of the common symptoms their patients experience.

**Silent airway reflux is the number one cause of the enigmatic chronic cough.[1] Silent reflux is also one of the most underdiagnosed and undertreated medical conditions in America.**

A thirty-three-year-old female Broadway star came to see me with a six-week history of change in her singing voice, post-nasal drip, sinusitis, chronic throat clearing, and cough. These symptoms were adversely affecting her ability to sing. Her RSI was 25, but she had never had heartburn.

Her examination and reflux testing revealed that she had severe reflux but her reflux pattern was exclusively nocturnal; that is, she refluxed only at night while she slept. But while the reflux happened at night, she experienced distressing voice symptoms during the day.

I placed her on *famotidine 20 mg* before dinner and bed as well as an *induction (detox) reflux diet* (chapter 6) with alkaline water, no alcohol, and no eating within four hours of bed. Her singing was back to normal within two weeks.

**Why is it that silent reflux patients don't have esophageal symptoms? It turns out that it takes a lot of reflux to damage the esophagus, but very little reflux can damage the more sensitive throat, sinuses, lungs, and vocal cords. That may be why people with silent reflux do not experience classic heartburn.**

The term *silent reflux* originated in 1987.[67] Dr. Walter Bo, a medical school colleague, was my patient. He had terrible morning hoarseness from nighttime reflux, because he habitually ate dinner very late and fell asleep on the sofa. He would then reflux all night.

I tried explaining his diagnosis, but Walter repeatedly denied having reflux because he thought heartburn and reflux were the same thing. When I clarified that he could have reflux without heartburn—as in his case when it occurred during sleep—Walter rolled his eyes and exclaimed, "I see. I have the silent kind of reflux." "Yes, Walter, that's it," I affirmed, "You have *silent reflux!*"

Unfortunately, when most people with silent airway reflux symptoms see their primary care physicians, they are incorrectly told they don't have reflux, or they are sent to a GI specialist. Since the medical specialties are broken down by anatomic parts of the body, specialists have limited knowledge of reflux that can affect different parts of the body, such as sinuses, throat, lungs, and esophagus.

The esophagus is usually treated by gastroenterologists, the throat and sinuses are usually treated by ear, nose, and throat specialists (otolaryngologists), and the trachea and lungs are usually treated by lung specialists (pulmonologists). All can be affected by silent airway reflux, but very few specialists can diagnose and treat it.

**Only a reflux specialist who knows what to look for in all affected areas and who has the right diagnostic tests is equipped to give you an accurate diagnosis.**

Otherwise, the doctor may guess wrong and treat you for an illness that you don't have. Symptoms of silent reflux can sometimes be caused by other diseases, which doctors may try to treat unsuccessfully, leaving you miserable, frustrated, and wasting money on unnessessary tests and drugs.

## Why Does Reflux Have So Many Names?

Why are there so many different labels for acid reflux? Because each specialist calls it by a different name. Furthermore, medical specialists are unaware of the literature and research in other specialties (hence the inclusion of the references in Appendix A).

## TABLE 5
# Common Medical Terms
# for Acid Reflux

GERD, or gastroesophageal reflux disease*

Reflux esophagitis or esophageal erosions

Extraesophageal reflux disease

Supraesophageal reflux disease

Heartburn or erosive esophagitis

LPR (Laryngopharyngeal reflux)**

Respiratory reflux

Esophageal reflux or Airway reflux

Atypical reflux disease

Barrett's esophagus

Esophageal reflux

Airway reflux

Silent reflux

.* This is the most often used medical term for esophageal reflux.
** This is the most often used medical term for respiratory or airway reflux

**Throughout this book, I prefer to use the terms *respiratory reflux* and *esophageal reflux*, which correspond with the more traditional terms *laryngopharyngeal reflux*, or LPR, and *gastroesophageal reflux disease*, or GERD.**

Respiratory and esophageal reflux are easier to pronounce and they make intuitive sense once you understand that the two types of reflux are in many ways—in symptoms and manifestations—quite different.

# The Reflux and Esophageal Cancer Epidemics

The prevalence of reflux—both esophageal reflux (GERD) and respiratory reflux (LPR)—has increased dramatically in our lifetimes.[2, 3, 81–86] A study published by ear, nose, and throat doctors showed that patient visits for airway reflux increased by almost 500 percent between 1990 and 2000.[83] Significantly, only 27 percent of the study patients were counseled about being on any kind of antireflux diet.[83]

**Since 1976, reflux has increased at a rate of 4 percent per year.[81] If you had $10 in 1976, at 4 percent compound interest, that money would be worth $40 today. Indeed, in 1976, 10 percent of Americans had reflux and now a whopping 40 percent have it. Reflux is epidemic![3]**

An even more ominous trend is the skyrocketing increase in the prevalence of esophageal cancer, which is caused by reflux.[84-86] The National Cancer Institute reports that esophageal cancer is the fastest growing cancer in the United States, having increased 850 percent since 1975.[3, 84] During this same period, its mortality rate also increased sevenfold, despite increased esophageal surveillance through more endoscopies.[3, 85, 86]

In addition, the prevalence of *Barrett's esophagus*, the precursor to esophageal cancer, is high. People with silent airway reflux, who have symptoms such as hoarseness, chronic cough, and sore throat, are just as likely to have Barrett's esophagus as people with esophageal reflux (GERD), having symptoms of heartburn and indigestion; the likelihood is about 8 percent for both groups.[77]

By the way, people who are worried about cancer deserve to be checked and the technology for this has changed. Doctors can now painlessly look inside while patients are awake using a technique called *transnasal esophagoscopy* (TNE).[21, 35, 40, 53, 65] Testing done with patients under sedation using older technology, such as *esophagogastroduodenoscopy* (EGD), is not recommended for people with airway reflux.

## Reflux Disease Is Now Common in Young People

Reflux used to be primarily a disease of overweight, middle-aged people. We now find that many reflux patients are neither obese nor older. Many are young and thin.

In 2010, we estimated the prevalence of airway and esophageal reflux in the United States by interviewing a geographically random sample of 656 US citizens.[3] People were asked all about their symptoms and medications. The data revealed that an astonishing 40 percent had reflux, 22 percent had esophageal reflux and another 18 percent had airway reflux.[3]

There were no significant differences between age, gender, and geographic region.[3] The most striking and unanticipated finding was that 37 percent of the twenty- to twenty-nine-year-old age group had reflux.

| TABLE 6 Prevalence of Reflux by Age Group | |
|---|---|
| 20–29 years | 37% |
| 30–39 years | 31% |
| 40–49 years | 43% |
| 50–59 years | 44% |
| 60–69 years | 41% |
| Over 70 years | 43% |

Why so many young people with reflux? According to the American Beverage Association, in 2010 the average twelve- to twenty-nine-year-old consumed 160 gallons of soft drinks[3]; that's a half-gallon of soft drinks per day, and the pH of those averages is 2.9 (the same as stomach acid).[2]

## Symptoms of Silent Airway Reflux

The symptoms and manifestations of reflux, silent airway reflux in particular, are so diverse that it is no wonder some people are skeptics. However, I have extensive experience and I believe I have seen every reflux-related scenario. Silent airway reflux can adversely affect any part of the aerodigestive tract; that is, all the breathing and eating passages. (See table 7 below and Chapter 9: Integrated Aerodigestive Medicine: A Healthcare Model for the Future.)

## TABLE 7

# Components of the Aerodigestive Tract

Nose, nasopharynx, and sinuses

Mouth, oropharynx, and pharynx

Hypopharynx and larynx

Trachea and lungs

Esophagus or esophageal body

Upper esophageal sphincter (UES)

Lower esophageal sphincter (LES)

Stomach and intestines

Reflux can be wholly responsible for any of the symptoms in table 8 below. But remember, one of the characteristics of silent airway reflux is that most sufferers have many symptoms, not just one—but not heartburn.

Besides chronic cough, the most common symptoms of silent airway reflux are chronic throat clearing, hoarseness, choking episodes, trouble swallowing, lump-in-the-throat sensation, shortness of breath, and asthma.[7, 67]

## TABLE 8

# Symptoms and Conditions Related to Reflux

| SYMPTOMS | CONDITIONS |
| --- | --- |
| Regurgitation | Dental caries and erosions |
| Chest pain | Esophageal spasm |
| Shortness of breath | Esophageal stricture |
| Choking episodes | Esophageal cancer |
| Hoarseness | Reflux laryngitis |
| Vocal fatigue | Throat cancer |
| Voice breaks | Sinusitis and allergic symptoms |
| Chronic throat clearing | Contact ulcers and granulomas |
| Excessive throat mucus | Asthma |
| Post-nasal drip | Sleep apnea |
| Chronic cough | Paroxysmal laryngospasm |
| Dysphagia | Globus pharyngeus |
| Difficulty swallowing | Laryngeal cancer |
| Difficulty breathing | Vocal cord dysfunction |
| Choking episodes | Paradoxical vocal cord movement |
| Lump-in-throat sensation | Vocal nodules and polyps |
| Food getting stuck | Pachydermia laryngitis |
| Airway obstruction | Recurrent leukoplakia |
| Wheezing | Polypoid degeneration |
| Heartburn | Idiopathic pulmonary fibrosis |
| | Chronic bronchitis |
| | Chronic obstructive lung disease |
| | Sudden infant death syndrome |
| | Laryngospasm |
| | Laryngomalacia |
| | Endotracheal intubation injury |

## The Diagnosis of Reflux-Related Cough

Let's return to the reflux symptom index (RSI) on page 13 and chronic cough index (CCI) on page 14. Your results should determine whether you are likely to have reflux-related cough. If your RSI is 15 or more and you have no heartburn, you have silent reflux. If your reflux-to-neurogenic ratio is 10:0, 9:1, or 8:2, your cough is due to airway reflux. In truth, you probably have reflux as a factor unless your R:N ratio is 2:8, 1:9, or 0:10. So what do you do after you self-diagnose?

You can beat reflux, but it is going to take work. You are going to have to make changes, and it's probably not going to be quick or easy. In addition, you will probably need to involve your doctor even if you are essentially self-treating (see Chapter 8: Don't Forget the Esophagus). And if you have post-nasal drip or a wet or productive cough, it will likely take months for all of your symptoms to disappear even after you get your reflux under control.

# 6
# DR. KOUFMAN'S REFLUX BOOT CAMP

I n my experience, reflux is not a chronic disease although most doctors think it is. I see it as a vicious spiral going downward. The more a person refluxes, the worse their esophageal valves work—and the worse their valves work, the more they reflux. The worse the reflux gets, the worse their esophageal function—and the worse their esophageal function, the worse their reflux gets. Figuratively, patients come see me when they are at the bottom, "in the dumpster," and they can't get out.

Before coming to see me many have already read my book *Dropping Acid: The Reflux Diet Cookbook & Cure* and modified their diets for the better, but they are still stuck. They need help and that's what I do.

The good news is that if you can completely stop reflux for two weeks, the system will usually recover. Sometimes it can be done with diet alone, but in many cases treatment requires medications to suppress acid or improve vagal and esophageal function. Fortunately, most airway reflux and esophageal reflux patients can become reflux free within six to twelve months.

This chapter cannot cover how and why I use every different treatment, because even after seeing perhaps as many as 200,000 reflux patients, I still view each person as a unique puzzle with a unique solution. That said, reflux treatment can generally be divided into three areas: (1) medical treatment (medications), (2) surgical treatment, and (3) treatment by dietary and lifestyle modifications.

## Medical Treatment

There are inexpensive, over-the-counter antacids like Tums and Rolaids that come packaged in a roll, like lifesavers, or in a bottle, and there are similar liquid antacid remedies like Maalox, Mylanta, and Gaviscon. The only antacid I recommend with any frequency is Gaviscon. Once ingested, it forms a "raft" that helps prevent reflux by blocking the stomach valve with a thick gel. Antacids are not used as a primary treatment in patients with airway reflux, and people who chronically self-treat heartburn with antacids should have a transnasal esophagoscopy to check for reflux-related esophageal damage.

The two main groups of acid-suppressive medications in current use are PPIs (*proton-pump inhibitors*) and H2As (*H2-antagonists*). PPIs and H2As both decrease acid production by inhibiting the acid-producing glands in the stomach, but there are fundamental differences between the two classes of drugs.

H2As like *cimetidine* (Tagamet) and *famotidine* (Pepcid) have few side effects and work better than PPIs for nighttime reflux. H2As are the drugs of choice for people who need to take antireflux medicine on an as-needed basis.

While PPIs such as omeprazole (Prilosec), esomeprazole (Nexium), lansoprazole (Prevacid), pantaprazole (Protonix), and others may be somewhat more powerful acid suppressives than H2As, PPIs have significant drawbacks and, in my opinion, should only be used under a doctor's supervision.

PPIs have many side effects including bloating, abdominal pain, and diarrhea, and are believed to be associated with osteoporosis (bone thinning and bone loss) and B12 deficiency. Furthermore, when PPIs are discontinued, many patients experience rebound, developing hyperacidity and recurrent reflux symptoms.

I believe that PPIs should not be sold over the counter, and when I prescribe PPIs I pair them with H2As and usually for a short period of time: weeks to months, not years. Furthermore, I never stop PPIs abruptly; I taper them and replace them with H2As to help weather the acid-rebound storm.

In addition to acid-suppressive drugs, there is another group of medications designed to improve esophageal function. So-called *prokinetic agents* improve esophageal motility (movement) and esophageal sphincter function. With the exception of gabapentin and domperidone, I rarely use any of the older prokinetics.

For a patient with severe nocturnal airway reflux with abnormal esophageal manometry, I may start by prescribing an induction reflux diet (see below) with no eating within five hours of bedtime, along with an H2A before lunch, dinner, and two before bedtime, and a prokinetic agent one to four times per day. Today, I often use gabapentin as a semi-prokinetic as this has special benefits for vagal function.

As the patient starts to improve, I discontinue the PPI first. With attention to dietary and lifestyle factors, most reflux patients can expect to be off all medication within six to twelve months.

The idea that people with esophageal reflux are different from those with airway reflux, or that they will need lifelong drug treatment is incorrect. In fact, there is reason to believe that the increasing rates of esophageal cancer may be related to the use of PPIs.

My belief is that PPIs provide symptomatic relief for many patients, particularly those with heartburn as their primary symptom, but the underlying disease continues to damage the esophagus. Taking a PPI so that you can eat whatever you want without heartburn is like sweeping dirt under the rug. At some point, it will catch up with you.

## Surgical Treatment

For patients who cannot get better even after an extended period of medication and reflux-clean living, surgery is an option. I see many of the most severe and recalcitrant refluxers, and only a small percent ever require surgery. In general, I tend to recommend surgery for younger patients with recalcitrant reflux and airway disease.

The type of surgery that I recommend is *laparoscopic fundoplication*.[50] This procedure involves wrapping the fundus (dome of the stomach) around the esophagus and then plicating (sewing) it to create a tight angle, a new valve, so that the stomach contents can't come back up, can't reflux.

Fundoplication surgery should be performed by an experienced surgeon who has performed at least two hundred to three hundred such procedures, and the wrap should be complete 360-degree wrap. This surgery can provide dramatic and permanent reflux relief when performed by the right surgeon.

## Dietary and Lifestyle Modifications

Globalization and urbanization have brought about dramatic changes in where, when, and what people eat. Fifty years ago, most people ate at home and prepackaged foods and beverages were uncommon.

Today, most big soft-drink and fast-food companies are global brands, and people everywhere are exposed to much higher levels of food additives than in previous generations. As the world's diet has become Americanized, reflux has followed.[2, 3]

Reflux is the disease of our civilization, and it is a great masquerader, quietly causing everything from tooth decay to nausea and sinusitis to asthma. It is estimated that 125 million Americans have reflux and half of them don't know it; it is estimated that there are 2 billion refluxing people worldwide.

The dramatic increases in reflux over the past forty years cannot be explained by the obesity epidemic alone. Coincident with the reflux epidemic, the world's diet has changed[2, 3] In our lifetimes, there have been four unhealthy dietary trends[2]:

1. Increased saturated fat
2. Increased high-fructose corn syrup
3. Increased exposure to organic pollutants (e.g., DDT, PCBs, dioxins)
4. Increased dietary acid (and other unhealthy additives)

The last of these trends, increased dietary acid, may hold the key to understanding the contemporary reflux epidemic and the dramatic increases in esophageal cancer.[2, 3]

## Excessive Dietary Acid Is the Missing Link

Why are reflux disease and esophageal cancer epidemic? Why, when esophageal cancer was relatively uncommon, did reflux patients usually present in middle age, while today we see comparable disease in patients in their twenties? Overacidity in the diet is the missing link, which explains the reflux epidemic and the increasing rates of Barrett's and esophageal cancer.[2, 3]

Following an outbreak of food poisoning in 1973, the US Congress mandated that the *Food and Drug Administration* (FDA) take responsibility for assuring the safety of processed food by establishing Good Manufacturing Practices.[2, 3] How was this accomplished? Through acidification of bottled and canned foods, which was intended to prevent bacterial growth and prolong shelf life.[2] From the 1979 Title 21 Act:

> Acidified foods should be so manufactured, processed, and packaged that a finished equilibrium pH value of 4.6 or below is achieved. If the finished equilibrium pH is 4.0 or below, then the measurement of acidity of the final product may be made by any suitable method.[2, 3]

Two generations later, the FDA continues this practice and has apparently never questioned whether acidification of the food supply might have potentially adverse health consequences. In other words, essentially by law the FDA demands that beverage and food manufacturers reduce the pH of products to the same pH (acidity) levels as stomach acid; bottled water is excepted.

In the United States, the arc of reflux and esophageal cancer epidemics appears to closely follow soft drink consumption. At the end of World War II, the average American consumed four eight-ounce soft drinks per week. In 2010, the average American between the ages of twelve and twenty-nine drank forty-nine eight-ounce soft drinks per week, an average of seven per day.[3] That number provided by the *American Beverage Association* averages almost two liters a day.

In addition to acid as a major food additive, the FDA allows over three hundred other chemicals to be added to food that are "generally regarded as safe" (GRAS).[2] Many of these GRAS food additives were grandfathered in during the 1970s without the benefit of contemporary state-of-the-art scientific scrutiny.[2] Thirteen percent of these additives are acids, and there is no evidence that the FDA (or anyone else) has ever studied the long-term effects of these GRAS, particulary acids.

Today, even organic baby food is acidified. We measured the pH of an organic banana baby food and found the pH to be 4.3. Normally, the pH of banana is about 5.7. But this so-called organic banana has added acid. Indeed, most bottled and canned foods and beverages are pH <4,[2] because phosphoric, acetic, ascorbic, and/or citric acids are added. Sometimes the food label may just read "vitamin C enriched or vitamin C enhanced."

In 1991, I published my magnum opus on reflux, which reviewed all that was known about the topic as well as my research on silent airway reflux.[7] It was written for membership in an academic society, the Triological Society. Similar to a doctoral thesis, I spent three years doing the research and writing, and to date, it is the most cited article in otolaryngology.

In the almost twenty-five years since its publication, the number of Americans with reflux disease has doubled.[1–3, 7, 81] In addition, when it comes to reflux diseases, particularly silent airway reflux, the medical establishment has been slow to accept new ideas.

**It is now clear that for airway reflux, the PPI-treatment failure rates are very high, regardless of dose. Acid-suppressive medications do not control reflux for most people, especially those with silent airway reflux. And, if the medication does help, should such patients have to stay on medication for life?**

The answer is *no*. For people with serious reflux, adjusting diet and lifestyle are essential for getting well.[2, 3] Remember, reflux begets worsening esophageal function, which in turn begets more reflux.

Thankfully, the opposite is also true, so that as inflammation and reflux improve, vavular and esophageal function improve and there is subsequently less reflux. Healthy function can be restored and diet and lifestyle are far more important than medication. However, for many patients with severe reflux, in the beginning, medication is needed as well as dietary and lifestyle changes.

Medication plus the two-week induction (detox) reflux diet greatly help by reducing acid and pepsin coming from below (the stomach), while reducing damaging acid (which activates pepsin) coming from above. In fact, today many of our reflux patients are being treated by diet alone, without medication.

## Evolution of the Induction (Detox) Reflux Diet

For more than twenty-five years, airway reflux patients in my practice were prescribed acid-suppressive medications as well as limited nutritional and lifestyle counseling. The latter consisted of a list of do's and don'ts (table 9).

---

**TABLE 9**

## Traditional Antireflux Diet and Lifestyle Modification Program

If you use tobacco, you must quit, because smoking causes reflux.

Don't wear clothing that is too tight, especially trousers, corsets, and belts.

Avoid exercising, especially weight-lifting, swimming, jogging, or yoga after eating.

Do not lie down just after eating and do not eat within three to four hours of bedtime.

Elevate the head of your bed if you are a nighttime refluxer (especially if you have morning hoarseness).

Limit your intake of red meat, butter, cheese, eggs, and anything with caffeine.

Completely avoid fried food, high-fat meats, onions, tomatoes, citrus fruit, fruit juice, carbonated beverages (soda), soft drinks, beer, liquor, wine, mints, and chocolate.

---

We recognized long ago that carbonated beverages, particularly caffeinated cola drinks, were a major risk factor for the development of airway reflux. Indeed, excessive consumption of carbonated beverages continues to be one of the most identified causes of reflux treatment failure among reflux patients.[2]

Based upon clinical experience, we also limited our patients' intake of citrus and hot (pepper) sauces. Other than those adjustments, the antireflux diet did not change very much until the last few years.

The cell biology of airway reflux helps explain why acid in foods and beverages causes so much trouble. Our landmark 2007 paper, "Activity/stability of human pepsin: Implications for reflux attributed laryngeal disease,"[62] showed that the enzyme pepsin was active up to pH 6.5. In addition, we also reported finding pepsin in the laryngeal biopsies of patients with airway reflux.[28, 46, 49]

Putting two and two together, we recognized that tissue-bound pepsin in the throats of airway refluxers could be activated by hydrogen ions (acids) from any source, including dietary acids.[2, 3]

It was pepsin that caused inflammation and tissue damage, and it required acid for activation. Consequently, we began to measure the pH of common foods and beverages, and to restrict consumption of anything known to be acidic for our reflux patients for a trial period of two weeks.

In 2008, as a consequence of finding acid in almost every common food and beverage,[2] we began to more strictly limit the acid intakes of our airway reflux patients, with outstanding results. As we measured the pH of more and more foods, the induction (detox) reflux diet evolved. Soon we had lists of good and bad foods and beverages.

In the ensuing years, we refined the induction reflux diet to exclude recognized reflux trigger foods as well as anything pH<5.[2, 3] The basic elements of the induction reflux diet in its present form are shown in table 10, and table 11 provides a complete list of the acceptable foods for the induction diet.

**TABLE 10**

# The Two-Week Induction Reflux Diet in a Nutshell

Grilled/baked/broiled/boiled fish, shellfish, and poultry

All vegetables (except onions, tomatoes, garlic, and peppers)

Breads, rice, grains, low-sugar cereals, oatmeal, and tofu

Melons, bananas, ginger, Manuka honey, chamomile tea

Low-fat soy, almond, or cow milk, alkaline water pH>8

One cup of coffee or caffeinated tea per day

No alcohol, soft drinks, or eating within four hours of bed

**TABLE 11**

# Induction Reflux Diet:
# What You Can Eat

Agave

Artificial sweetener
(max. 2 packets per day)

Bagels and (non-fruit) low-fat
muffins

Banana (great snack food)

Beans (black, red, lima, lentils)

Bread (especially whole grain and
rye)

Caramel (max. 4 tablespoons per
week)

Celery (great snack food)

Chamomile tea (other herbal teas
are not acceptable)

Chicken (grilled/broiled/baked/
steamed; no skin)

Chicken stock or bouillon

Coffee (max. one cup per day;
best with milk)

Egg whites

Fennel

Fish (including shellfish, grilled,
broiled, baked, steamed)

Ginger (ginger root,
powdered or preserved)

Graham crackers

Herbs (excluding all peppers, citrus,
garlic, and mustard)

Honey (Manuka honey preferred)

Low-fat milk (cow, soy, or almond
milk)

Melon (honeydew, cantaloupe,
watermelon)

Mushrooms (raw or cooked)

Oatmeal (all whole-grain cereals)

Olive oil (max. 2 tablespoons per
day)

Parsley

Popcorn (plain or salted, no butter)

Potatoes (all of the root vegetables
except onions)

Rice (healthy, especially brown rice,
a staple during induction)

Soups (homemade with noodles
and low-acid veggies)

Tofu

Turkey breast (organic, no skin)

Vegetables (raw or cooked, but no
onions, tomatoes, garlic, or
peppers)

Vinaigrette (max. 1 teaspoon per
day; you must toss salads)

Whole-grain breads, crackers, and
breakfast cereals

I previously reported successful results of the induction reflux diet in twenty patients with recalcitrant (PPI-medication-resistant) airway reflux.[3] All twenty claimed excellent compliance with the diet, and 95 percent (19 out of 20) improved. Three subjects became completely asymptomatic, and another went from an initial RSI (reflux symptom index) of 28 to a post-diet RSI of 4.

The mean pre-diet RSI was 14.8 and the mean post-diet RSI was 8.6 ($P=0.023$); the mean RSI improvement was 6.3 points. The mean pre-diet RFS[3] (reflux-finding score) was 12.0, and the mean post-diet RFS was 8.3 ($P<0.001$).[3] In a word, these differences, before and after low-acid diet, were highly statistically significant. And don't forget, these were patients who had not experienced any relief from their reflux on high-dose (twice-daily) PPIs, the most powerful medication.

## Four Phases of the Reflux Diet

There are four phases of the reflux diet: (1) induction, (2) transition, (3) maintenance, and (4) longevity. To reiterate, the purpose of the two-week induction reflux diet is to wash out pepsin and restore more normal functioning of antireflux defenses.

The induction reflux diet has been the cornerstone of my dietary and lifestyle program for patients with both airway and esophageal reflux. An additional adjunctive therapy that has been added within the last few years is alkaline water.

We evaluated a natural artesian alkaline (pH 8.8) water (Evamor™) in the laboratory and found that it instantaneously and permanently denatured (killed) pepsin; it also had good buffering capacity.[68] Many of my patients report that alkaline water is a key variable in their recovery.

The induction reflux diet is still recommended for just the first two weeks with a gradual reintroduction of some additional fatty foods and other historically refluxogenic foods. Cheese, eggs, meats, sauces, and condiments are allowed in moderation as flavorings, but all phases of the reflux diet remain relatively low-acid (not no-acid) and low-fat (not no-fat).

We teach patients moderation, particularly with fatty foods, using tasty fats as flavorings rather than as main ingredients. We also introduce the concept of *pH balancing* in which acidic foods may be combined with non-acidic foods. Acidic fruits, for example, that are not allowed by themselves, may be fine if added to breakfast cereal with high-pH milk (preferably low-fat milk) or if consumed along with alkaline water.

Finally, during the induction reflux diet, no eating is allowed within four hours of bed. Even eating healthy food too late in the evening can be a problem. It actually takes four hours for the stomach to empty completely. After the induction, the time between eating and recumbency (lying down) can be three hours.

A patient of mine was a restaurant manager who got off work at eleven at night and after eating a big dinner, would go to bed by midnight. Despite taking reflux medication, he suffered terrible heartburn every morning, and sometimes during the night as well.

When I explained that he didn't have a chance of beating his reflux as long as he was eating dinner before bed, he replied, "I knew you were going to say that. I guess I am going to have to make some big changes?" "Not really," I told him. "Just take a break to have your dinner before eight."

Night eating is a major cause of silent airway reflux. It is also a major risk factor for obesity, diabetes, hypertension, snoring, and sleep apnea. Most people who go to bed with a full stomach are going to reflux, and lying on the sofa after dinner has the same effect. Actually, the best thing a person can do after dinner is to take a walk. Even after induction, night eating is one of the most common causes of both airway and esophageal reflux.

Based upon many years of examining pH-monitoring data, we know that most patients with mild to moderate airway reflux are upright (daytime) refluxers, often with many relatively short periods of acid/pepsin exposure. In contrast, patients with severe airway reflux and breathing problems are typically supine (nocturnal) refluxers, with acid/pepsin contact times (reflux episodes) that can be hours long each night.

Prolonged reflux results in much more severe tissue inflammation and damage. Indeed, a single two- to six-hour supine nocturnal reflux event can produce hoarseness, sore throat, and cough symptoms that can last several weeks.

After induction, there is *transition,* phase two. This phase requires trial and error as foods and beverages are reintroduced. I usually start by adding back egg yolks, condiments, some fruits that are relatively low-acid, such as berries, pears, and red apples, and some meats that are relatively low-fat, such as white pork and lean beef.

Three-egg omelets can be made with just one yolk as an example of low-fat rather than no-fat eating, and for meats, portion control is important. Patients are instructed to order all dressings, condiments, cheeses, and sauces on the side so they can add them themselves and thus consume relatively small amounts. Wine and cocktails may be added back, but only one drink per day, and not too late in the evening.

During the transition phase, which can last months, there must be experimentation with different foods. The truth is that everyone with reflux is different, and even foods that are forbidden during the induction phase may be well tolerated by some individuals, including onions, tomatoes, garlic, and peppers. These are all *idio-syncratic foods*; that is, some patients can tolerate one but not another, and some are better tolerated cooked than raw, such as tomatoes and onions. Some people can tolerate garlic flavorings but not garlic itself, and so on.

It is also important to point out that people have different *trigger foods*, which are foods that cause symptoms, sometimes immediate symptoms, such as throatburn, or delayed symptoms, even a day later. Items on the best-for-reflux food list can be trigger foods for some people.

The key endpoints of the transition phase are fewer symptoms and improvement on the laryngeal examination. I have used the reflux-finding score (RFS) for every reflux patient at every visit and the RFS should be lower (closer to normal) as time passes. In addition, during transition I attempt to ween patients off antireflux medications, especially PPIs.

H2As, such as famotidine 20 mg, can be used up to four times a day (before each meal and at bedtime) without problems. Furthermore, H2As are acceptable as *ad hoc* medications, taken as needed.

In addition, H2As should be preemptively taken before dinner and before bed if you know that you are going to be eating later than usual or eating foods that may be a problem. The same is not true of PPIs that are often associated with rebound hyperacidity after they are discontinued.

During the third phase, *maintenance*, you can sustain a healthy lifestyle with reflux under control for a prolonged period. At this point, you should be able to comfortably eat in restaurants, and feel that healthy eating is easy.

I call the fourth and final phase *longevity*, when you have no reflux, when you are no longer on reflux medication, when you are near your ideal body weight, and you can effortlessly eat at home or dine out without fearing reflux.

Does this sound too good to be true? Longevity takes work and persistence, and sometimes the help of a nutritionist. But, normal physiology can be reestablished in most refluxers with outstanding long-term outcomes. This is proof that reflux is a disease of what we eat and when we eat it.

In summary, excessive acid and fat in the diet, late-night eating, and consumption of soft drinks and alcohol are the most important and reversible lifestyle-related factors contributing to the development of airway and esophageal reflux. With customized dietary and lifestyle modifications, most reflux patients can be managed successfully. Without such changes, all other treatments are doomed to failure.

One final note: From a public health point of view, it would be very beneficial to mandate that pH (acidity) of all bottled and canned foods and beverages be printed on nutritional labels. This would help people with reflux make informed choices.

# 7

# ASTHMA THAT ISN'T ASTHMA

According to the Centers for Disease Control, one in twelve Americans (8 percent) has asthma, and 17 percent of poor, non-white children.[87] But is asthma the correct diagnosis?[1, 88, 89]

Of the patients who come to me with a diagnosis of asthma, only 20 percent have it, with four out of five having been misdiagnosed.[1] These *pseudo-asthmatics* never experienced *expiratory wheezing* or benefitted from asthma treatment.

This huge misdiagnosed group actually had *inspiratory stridor* and *reactive airway disease* caused by airway reflux. Such include *laryngospasm* and *paradoxical vocal cord movement*.[66] What is the difference between reflux-caused pseudo-asthma and the real thing?

**If you, or someone you know has asthma, ask this question: "When you have trouble breathing, do you have more trouble getting air *in* (during inspiration) or *out* (during expiration)?" If the answer is *in*, it's reflux, and if the answer is *out*, it's asthma.**

The problem is that the lung doctors who rely on breathing tests called *pulmonary function tests* (PFTs) are often fooled by the results, because patients with reflux-related reactive airway disease may show some improvement on PFTs after *bronchodilators* (used for asthma) are administered. All forms of reactive airways disease, including airway reflux and asthma may improve to some degree with certain types of inhalers, such as *albuterol*.

How do I know that most of the asthma patients coming to see me actually have reflux and not asthma? In addition to having no history of expiratory wheezing and little or no significant response to asthma treatment, these patients have all the findings of airway reflux; they have dreadful reflux-testing results; *and* they respond to reflux treatment.

In my unpublished research paper discussed earlier, the mean reflux symptom index of the pseudo-asthma subgroup was 25, which is quite high.[1] That means that those patients, previously diagnosed as asthmatics, also had other symptoms such as hoarseness, globus, dysphagia, excess throat mucus, etc. (see the reflux symptom index, page 13).

In addition, my pseudo-asthma group had an average of 123 reflux episodes into the throat according to high-definition airway pH monitoring.[1] By any criteria, that is a lot of pharyngeal (throat) reflux! Those patients were treated for reflux and almost all got well; although five did need to have *antireflux surgery*. (In the remaining few, the most common reasons for treatment failure were uncontrolled reflux, patient noncompliance, and other complicating concurrent diagnoses.)

If my data are in any way suggestive of the magnitude of misdiagnosis of asthma in the general population, then as a public service, let me reiterate five key points:

1. Asthma is associated with difficulty getting air *out*, with exhalation (wheezing), while difficulty getting air *in* is reactive airway disease due to airway reflux.
2. Patients with airway reflux usually have many symptoms that suggest airway reflux, including hoarseness, shortness of breath, post-nasal drip, too much throat mucus, cough, difficulty swallowing, and a sensation of a lump in the throat.
3. Physicians unable to examine the larynx and throat or not

familiar with the findings of airway reflux should send the patient to a clinician who can make a proper diagnosis.

4. Physicians should recognize that when asthma patients do not respond to asthma treatment, reflux may be the alternative diagnosis.

5. Treatment for chronic cough patients with reflux and reactive airways disease requires major dietary and lifestyle modifications, and in this group, antireflux surgery (*fundoplication*) may be recommended.

And I'll add one more:

6. The single most important therapeutic intervention for childhood and adult "asthma" (airway reflux) may be *no bedtime snacks!*

Effective long-term reflux treatment has saved such patients from lung transplants, and I have watched many patients with chronic bronchitis and COPD (modestly) recover lung function after months or years of tight reflux control highlighted by healthy eating and living.

**I have treated patients with all kinds of lung diseases who have had reflux for decades, and I firmly believe that 70 percent of lung disease is due to or complicated by airway reflux. If I am right, this represents a colossal paradigm shift in medicine.**

In the last decade, one of the most interesting breakthroughs in understanding the relationship between reflux and lung disease occurred in the transplant world. Lung transplant failure is not due to organ rejection; it is because of reflux![88]

Reflux is the cause of lung transplant failure to such an extent that some transplant programs now recommend antireflux surgery before lung transplantation.[88] (I suggest the same surgery for my patients whose airway reflux is causing lung disease—just twenty-five years sooner.)

I believe that most people who need lung transplants have reflux. Indeed, idiopathic pulmonary fibrosis is probably wholly or in part due to reflux, and the same is true for COPD (chronic obstructive lung disease) and for all forms of reactive airway disease as well. Again, based upon years of clinical experience, I believe that roughly 70 percent of lung disease is reflux related.

Interestingly, using a pepsin assay, one of my research colleagues, Nikki Johnston, and her group at the Medical College of Wisconsin have reported that 72 percent (47 out of 65) of the lung secretion samples of children with chronic cough, wheezing, and recurrent pneumonia were pepsin positive.[89] In other words, they demonstrated conclusive airway reflux in 72 percent of the respiratory disease children that they studied.[89]

In summary, people who have airway reflux and trouble breathing all deserve an accurate diagnosis, and prolonged and aggressive reflux control when indicated. In addition, all forms of reactive airway disease are mediated by the vagus nerve, so therapy directed at improving vagal function may potentially be important for both chronic cough and pseudo-asthma. Of course, there is some overlap, with people who have both reactive airway disease from reflux and asthma. There is often a large neurogenic component to reactive airway disease, including choking episodes (e.g., laryngospasm), *vocal cord dysfunction*, paradoxical vocal cord movement, and asthma.

# 8
# DON'T FORGET THE ESOPHAGUS

One of the most common questions I am asked is "What happens if long-term reflux goes untreated?" The answer is that serious and life-threatening complications are possible, and the likelihood is increasing. As a matter of fact, even with daily proton-pump inhibitor treatment (such as Prilosec, Nexium, "purple pills"), deadly complications such as *esophageal cancer* can still occur.

The prevalence of esophageal and throat cancer is on the rise. In fact, cancer of the esophagus—known to be caused by esophageal reflux—is the fastest growing cancer in the United States, up a whopping 850 percent since the 1970s.[3, 84]

If you have long-standing reflux (esophageal or airway reflux), you should have a throat and esophageal examination. Believe it or not, this may mean seeing two different doctors because not all ENT doctors (otolaryngologists) perform esophagoscopy, and very few GIs perform *laryngoscopy* or throat examinations.

**Your best choice for obtaining a comprehensive examination is an ENT doctor who performs transnasal esophagoscopy (TNE).**[21, 40, 53, 65]

I have been performing these examinations (throat and esophagus) at the same time for many years.

In reviewing my chronic cough cases, I was surprised to find that 64 percent had esophageal disease.[1] The findings were *esophagitis* 48 percent, *hiatal hernia* 18 percent, *candida* (fungal) *esophagitis* 8 percent, Barrett's esophagus (esophageal precancer) 8 percent, and one had *esophageal varices*.[1]

My chronic cough study group may or may not accurately represent the general population because the average duration of chronic cough symptoms in my patients was ten years.[1] Nevertheless, the data strongly suggest that patients with silent airway reflux, essentially all refluxers, undergo throat *and* esophageal examinations. However, the idea that you can only be checked for cancer in a special facility and under anesthesia is archaic.

**Since early detection is vital to improve esophageal cancer survival, routine esophageal screening using transnasal esophagoscopy (TNE) is recommended for people with both airway and esophageal reflux. TNE is by far the safest and most cost-effective as the first esophageal examination method.[65]**

TNE is performed with the patient seated comfortably in a chair using an ultrathin *endoscope* that is introduced though the nose and then easily advanced all the way down into the stomach. TNE exam is comfortable, the examination images are superior, and accurately obtained biopsies may be performed when needed.

*Esophagogastroduodenoscopy* (EGD) performed by the gastroenterologist is the wrong type of esophageal examination for patients with reflux. Since EGD is done with the patient sedated, the esophagus is collapsed, and once the first cup-forceps biopsy is taken, there is blood in the field. Thus, errors in diagnosis may result from errors in tissue sampling.

The finding of columnar (stomach) lining in a biopsy obtained during EGD does not translate to a diagnosis of Barrett's esophagus. And Barrett's esophagus is not a diagnosis that people want to have since it is a known precursor to esophageal cancer. In the past, people with Barrett's were told that they had a one percent per year chance of getting cancer. Today, we believe that the risk is much less than that and that Barrett's can be healed with a long-term low-acid, low-fat diet.[69]

Here's an interesting and important case example:

A patient from Seattle came to see me. She had been enrolled in the Seattle Barrett's Program, having been positively diagnosed by biopsy with Barrett's esophagus. After she read my book, *Dropping Acid: The Reflux Diet Cookbook & Cure*, she put herself on my strict reflux diet (table 11, page 50) for a full year.

So after a year on the induction reflux diet, she came to see me and asked that I perform TNE. I did, and her Barrett's was gone.[69] Paradigm shift: Barrett's esophagus reversed with low-acid diet and alkaline water!

In the last few years, I have seen a trend in the overdiagnosis of Barrett's esophagus in patients undergoing EGD. Less than half of the patients who came to me having already received a diagnosis of Barrett's esophagus from EGD actually had it. Since TNE is performed with the patient awake and swallowing normally, it is easier to see the normal anatomic landmarks so that more accurate biopsies can be obtained.

**In summary, the diagnosis of respiratory reflux is *not* made by *endoscopy* (TNE or otherwise), but by clinical diagnosis, laryngeal findings, and by airway reflux testing. *However*, once the diagnosis of airway reflux is made, an esophageal examination (TNE) is indicated to rule out significant esophageal disease.**

# 9

# INTEGRATED AERODIGESTIVE MEDICINE: A HEATHCARE MODEL FOR THE FUTURE

Any person with an enigmatic chronic cough will tell you that the specialist model of American medicine has failed. In truth, it has failed for a large number of patients and at many different levels. Not only do we have too many specialists, but too many practice so narrow a specialty that often patients receive incorrect, expensive, and wasteful medical care.

An illustration of the chronic cough patient's predicament with the specialist model of American medicine is the elephant in the fable of the three blind men and the elephant.

> The first blind man, feeling the leg of the elephant, exclaims, "I can see it clearly; the elephant is like a big tree." The second blind man holds the trunk and says, "No, the elephant is like a very large snake." The third blind man grasps an ear. "You are both wrong," he proclaims. "The elephant is really like a gigantic leaf." Each blind man embraces a part of the truth, but none understands its entirety.

In the case of chronic cough, the three blind men are the three medical specialties: (1) the otolaryngologist (ENT, the ear, nose, and throat physician); (2) the gastroenterologist (GI physician); and (3) the pulmonologist (PUL, chest and lung specialist).

The problem is not just ignorance. Today, many doctors behave more like entrepreneurs than healers. Each "profit center" attempts to maximize income by manipulating the medical billing and coding system. Indeed, most medical professional societies offer their physicians advanced training in coding so that they can effectively maximize income.

It is worse than you think. Today in many hospitals, coding specialists routinely make patient-care rounds with the doctors to insure that no code goes unbilled. The idea is that hospitals want to absolutely maximize possible income. And, yes, they stretch the truth a lot every day to do so.

## Corruption Is Why Healthcare Is So Expensive

**The needs of patients have been lost in a healthcare system dominated by for-profit corporate medicine characterized by collusion, price fixing, and corruption.**

In 2012, I had back surgery, a L3-L4-L5 fusion. I now have two titanium plates and six screws in my back. The hospital billed $111,000 for the hardware alone; unbelievably, it actually was $15,000 per screw. (I know for a fact that you can purchase an excellent quality titanium screw at Home Depot for under a dollar.)

The punch line is not that the hospital billed so outrageously, but that my insurance company paid them $146,000 for my surgery ($99,000 for the hardware) and that didn't cover professional fees. My surgeon charged $117,000, and I believe that he received payment of $104,000. Meanwhile, I am still being billed by the hospital and the surgeon; both want more money.

The total bill for the surgery was $260,000. In some European countries, comparable surgery costs about $10,000. One might reasonably ask where the other $250,000 went.

Returning to chronic cough and reflux, there is corruption in endoscopy. Many doctors have profound conflicts of interest because of *ambulatory surgery centers*. ASCs are big business. Typically, a doctor negotiates an ownership position in an ASC with the understanding that she or he will perform a certain number of procedures, say a thousand per year, at that ASC. Conflict of interest? The return on investment is astonishing! One GI from New York happily informed me that the annual income from his ASC was over $1 million.

Last year, there were 10 million sedated endoscopies performed in the United States at a *facilities fee* cost of $10 billion; that is, an average of $1,000 per procedure. And that does not include the professional fees of the gastroenterologist, anesthesiologist, and pathologist.

Also questionable, when GIs perform *upper endoscopy* for reflux, they routinely examine the entire upper GI tract and perform biopsies. Why? Is it because EGD (esophagogastroduodenoscopy) with biopsy pays much more than a lesser procedure or a procedure without biopsies?

When it comes to non-pulmonary chronic cough, pulmonologists also appear to be inefficient and wasteful. When a patient sees a pulmonologist with any type of reactive airway disease or shortness of breath, the doctor will usually perform pulmonary function tests (PFTs). She or he may also perform *bronchoscopy*, endoscopy of the airway and lungs, but these doctors are not trained to examine the throat. When it comes to silent airway reflux, the usual result is misdiagnosis and incorrect treatment.

Most pulmonologists diagnose asthma in all cases of reactive airway disease, because they apparently cannot differentiate inspiratory, airway reflux-caused reactive airway disease from true asthma characterized by expiratory wheezing. The misdiagnosis of asthma is costly. No one knows exactly how much; however, asthma medication alone costs over $50 billion annually in the United States. See Chapter 7: Asthma That Isn't Asthma.

Otolaryngologists should be able to examine the larynx (voice box) and throat, but they are generally handicapped by outmoded instrumentation and inadequate training. Thus, most ENTs can neither accurately diagnose nor effectively treat airway reflux.

Perhaps the greatest waste due to inaccurate diagnosis in the otolaryngology area is sinusitis. Many patients come to me after having had multiple unsuccessful sinus surgeries, still suffering the same symptoms. Yes, again it's airway reflux. Nocturnal (nighttime) reflux in particular can cause sinus symptoms, the most common of which is *post-nasal drip*.

The typical chronic cough patient who comes to see me has been coughing for more than a decade and has already seen more than a dozen physicians (ENTs, GIs, PULs, allergists, etc.). One patient who had been coughing for twenty years reported that he had seen thirty-four doctors, some from four major medical centers, before seeing me.

## Restructuring Healthcare

Where did this excessive, inefficient, and unnecessarily expensive medical mess come from? The healthcare industry has shown a strong propensity to chase funding. When Medicare agreed to cover renal dialysis, for example, new dialysis centers quickly sprung up everywhere.

Remember, US healthcare is private industry, but much of it is paid for by the government, e.g., Medicare, Medicaid. A big part of the problem is lack of accountability—there is little or no objective scrutiny in healthcare. What do we get for our money? Fifteen-thousand-dollar-a-piece screws?

Specialist medicine has proliferated in part because Americans want to have the "best." They like seeing the best doctors just as they like seeing the best sports teams. The problem, however, is what doctor to see when your self-diagnosis is wrong? The best at what?

Furthermore, while the idea of seeing the "best doctor" is appealing, there is no such doctor when it comes to non-pulmonary chronic cough, silent airway reflux, and *vagally mediated* neurogenic syndromes.

Today, people are skeptical and cautious, and at this point consumer confidence cannot be restored by the marketing claim that "We are the best." Patients are rightly mistrustful of the current healthcare system.

**People no longer believe that healthcare providers necessarily have their best interests at heart. It is now clear that patients must be their own advocates and that for-profit medicine leads to more attention to gain and less to quality patient care.**

We pay two to four times more than any other developed country for healthcare, and we rank thirty-seventh in quality of care. Last year, the price tag for US healthcare was $2.7 trillion.* Strip away the excesses and the price would probably have been closer to $700 billion ($0.7 trillion). That's a lot of excess!

We need a healthcare system that is less fragmented and self-serving. Specialists often do what they do well, but nothing more.

If chronic cough, airway reflux, reactive airway disease, and (vagal) neurogenic syndromes are so prevalent—almost one-out-of-five (18 percent) Americans has airway reflux[3] and falls into one of the above

---

* Elisabeth Rosenthal, "The $2.7 Trillion Medical Bill," *New York Times*, June 1, 2013.

categories—then the current system is wasting massive healthcare dollars on inappropriate diagnostics and ineffective treatments.

**Maybe we don't need so many gastroenterologists, pulmonologists, and otolaryngologists. Maybe we need doctors who take better care of the whole patient with aerodigestive diseases. Reflux is the tip of an appalling iceberg.**

## Integrated Aerodigestive Medicine

I have practiced *integrated aerodigestive medicine* for thirty years now. What does that mean? I am part otolaryngologist, but I know the parts of otolaryngology that most otolaryngologists don't know. I am part gastroenterologist, but I know the parts of gastroenterology that most gastroenterologists don't know. And I am part pulmonologist, but I know the parts of pulmonology that most pulmonologists don't know.

I don't practice all aspects of aerodigestive medicine, and I know my limitations. I have almost nothing to do with the liver, colon, heart, teeth, sinuses, etc.

I am an expert in the vagal system, and that includes the whole airway and the whole digestive tract. And, yes, all of these parts are connected anatomically and functionally.

As I have become well known as an airway reflux expert, with expertise in non-medical treatment (namely, diet and lifestyle), more and more patients with esophageal reflux (GERD) have come to see me.

A common story is "I had endoscopy, and I was told that I had Barrett's esophagus. I was given a pill and told to come back in a year." Apparently, most GIs think that the only treatment for reflux, no matter how severe, is a purple pill (PPI).

Unlike anatomic (organ-specific) medical specialties, integrated aerodigestive medicine is system driven and symptom driven. It combines elements of all the overlapping aerodigestive tract medical specialties with a special focus on the diagnosis and treatment of airway reflux. Further, as a preventative approach to wellness, integrated aerodigestive medicine emphasizes dietary health, lifestyle education, and behavior modification.

The aerodigestive tract must be treated as a unified system for which physicians are trained. In addition, precision diagnostics (e.g., laryngeal electromyography, airway reflux testing) are the key

---

**TABLE 12**

# Aerodigestive Symptoms

| | |
|---|---|
| Allergies | Indigestion |
| Asthma | Laryngitis |
| Burning tongue | Laryngospasm |
| Chest pain (non-cardiac) | Nausea |
| Choking episodes | Painful speaking (odynophonia) |
| Chronic cough | Paradoxical vocal cord movement |
| Chronic throat clearing | Post-nasal drip |
| COPD (chronic obstructive pulmonary disease) | Regurgitation |
| Dental and gum disease | Shortness of breath |
| Difficulty swallowing | Sinusitis |
| Excessive throat mucus | Sleep apnea |
| Food getting stuck | Throatburn |
| Globus (a lump-in-throat sensation) | Vocal cord dysfunction |
| Heartburn | Vocal fatigue |
| Hoarseness | Vocal nodules and polyps |
| | Voice breaks |
| | Wheezing |

to accurate diagnosis, and at present, few physicians perform any, let alone all of them.

So if integrated aerodigestive medicine is a new "specialty," who should see such a physician, and for what? Shown on page 69 is a list of common integrated aerodigestive medicine symptoms.

The idea that people with these symptoms need to be seen by a committee of different specialists, one for each problem, makes no sense, particularly since reflux and vagal dysfunction are responsible for most.

**For people who don't have chronic cough but have another reflux-related or neurogenic symptom, you could read this book by substituting painful speaking or burning throat for chronic cough and the information and approach will still be relevant.**

A doctor practicing integrated aerodigestive medicine, as I do, must have certain skills and diagnostic technology:

1. Ability to obtain and interpret high-definition examination of the nose and throat (transnasal videostroboscopy) with still imaging
2. Ability to calculate an accurate reflux-finding score
3. Ability to diagnose subtle vocal cord paresis
4. High-definition esophageal manometry
5. Ambulatory, double-probe, 24-hour (simultaneous esophageal and pharyngeal) pH monitoring
6. Laryngeal electromyography
7. Transnasal esophagoscopy
8. Pulmonary function testing

Let's remember, the vagus nerve is the nerve of the entire aerodigestive tract. I am a doctor of the vagus, and therefore I am a doctor of the aerodigestive tract. I do not, however, practice medicine in a vacuum. I have a team of colleagues to whom I refer when appropriate.

It is a big team because I understand that I have limitations. I am not a sinus surgeon and sometimes one is needed; I am not a pulmonologist and sometimes one is needed, and so forth. No less than twenty-five stacks of business cards sit on my windowsill for those colleagues to whom I refer patients. They form a network designed to enable me to provide comprehensive care for my patients.

---

**TABLE 13**

## Aerodigestive Medicine Team

Acupuncture

Allergy

Audiology

Cardiology

Dentistry

Endocrinology

Gastroenterology

General surgery (for antireflux surgery)

Internal medicine

Otolaryngology

Psychiatry

Pulmonology

Speech-language pathology

I refer to all of those professionals as appropriate, but I remain in charge of the overall health and well-being of my patients. I am the quarterback of the team. I call the plays and I insure that we doctors communicate for the benefit of our patients.

In the future, residency programs in integrated aerodigestive medicine will focus on chronic cough and other aerodigestive symptoms with the understanding that reflux plays a huge role in the severity of disease, and that environmental, dietary, infectious, neurogenic, inflammatory, and emotional factors act together. All must be considered as part of the problem, and the solution should be seen as unique for each individual patient.

In my opinion, a major overhaul of the healthcare system is needed. Health is not a commodity and should never be treated as such. Restructuring the American healthcare system will require a compassionate and uncorporate new paradigm. Integrated aerodigestive medicine provides an excellent model of efficient restructuring.

# APPENDIX A:
# REFERENCES

1. Koufman J. The Diagnosis and Management of Non-Pulmonary Chronic Cough. Presented at the American Broncho-Esophagological Association annual meeting, April 19, 2012, San Diego CA. (Unpublished data, 2012)

2. Koufman J, Stern J, Bauer MM. *Dropping Acid: The Reflux Diet Cookbook & Cure*. Katalitix Media, New York, 2010.

3. Koufman JA. Low-Acid Diet for Recalcitrant Laryngopharyngeal Reflux: Therapeutic Benefits and Their Implications. Ann Otol Rhinol Laryngol 120:281–87, 2011.

4. Little FB, Koufman JA, Kohut RI, Marshal RB. Effect of gastric acid on the pathogenesis of subglottic stenosis. Ann of Otol Rhinol Laryngol 94:516–19, 1985.

5. Koufman JA, Wiener GJ, Wu WC, Castell DO. Reflux laryngitis and its sequelae: The diagnostic role of 24-hour pH monitoring. J Voice 2:78–89, 1988.

6. Weiner GJ, Koufman JA, Wu WC, Cooper JB, Richter JE, Castell DO. Chronic hoarseness secondary to gastroesophageal reflux disease: Documentation with 24-H ambulatory pH monitoring. Amer J Gastroenterol 84:12–18, 1989.

7. Koufman JA. The otolaryngologic manifestations of gastroesophageal reflux disease (GERD): A clinical investigation of 225 patients using ambulatory 24-hour pH monitoring and an experimental investigation of the role of acid and pepsin in the development of laryngeal injury. Laryngoscope 101(Suppl. 53):1–78, 1991.

8. Koufman JA. Aerodigestive manifestations of gastroesophageal reflux. What we don't yet know. Chest 104:1321–22, 1993.

9. Ott DJ, Ledbetter MS, Chen MYM, Koufman JA, Gelfand DW. Correlation of lower esophageal mucosal ring and 24-h pH monitoring of the esophagus. Amer J Gastroenterol 91:61–64, 1996.

10. Koufman JA, Sataloff RT, Toohill R. Laryngopharyngeal reflux: Consensus report. J Voice 10:215–16, 1996.

11. Loughlin CJ, Koufman JA. Paroxysmal laryngospasm secondary to gastroesophageal reflux. Laryngoscope 106:1502–5, 1996.

12. Loughlin CJ, Koufman JA, Averill DB, Cummins MM, Yong-Jae K, Little JP, Miller Jr. IJ, Meredith W. Acid-induced laryngospasm in a canine model. Laryngoscope 106:1506–9, 1996.

13. Koufman JA, Burke AJ. The etiology and pathogenesis of laryngeal carcinoma. Oto Clin N A 30:1–19, 1997.

14. Little JP, Matthews BL, Glock MS, Koufman JA, Reboussin DM, Loughlin CJ, McGuirt Jr. WF. Extraesophageal pediatric reflux: 24-hour double-probe pH monitoring of 222 children. Ann Otol Rhinol Laryngol Suppl 169:1–16, 1997.

15. Matthews BL, Little JP, McGuirt Jr. WF, Koufman JA. Reflux in infants with laryngomalacia: Results of 24-hour double-probe pH monitoring. Otolaryngol Head Neck Surg 120:860–64, 1999.

16. Koufman JA, Amin M, Panetti M. Prevalence of reflux in 113 consecutive patients with laryngeal and voice disorders. Otolaryngol Head Neck Surg 123:385–88, 2000.

17. Koufman JA, Postma GN, Whang C, Rees C, Amin M, Belafsky P, Johnson P, Connolly K, Walker F. Diagnostic laryngeal electromyography: The Wake Forest experience 1955–1999. Otolaryngol Head Neck Surg 124:603–6, 2001.

18. Amin MR, Koufman JA. Vagal neuropathy after upper respiratory infection: A viral etiology? Am J Otolaryngol 22:251–56, 2001.

19. Amin MR, Postma GN, Johnson P, Digges N, Koufman JA. Proton pump inhibitor resistance in the treatment of laryngopharyngeal reflux. Otolaryngol Head Neck Surg 125:374–78, 2001.

20. Duke SG, Postma GN, McGuirt Jr. WF, Ririe D, Averill DB, Koufman JA. Laryngospasm and diaphragmatic arrest in the immature canine after laryngeal acid exposure: A possible model for sudden infant death syndrome (SIDS). Ann Otol Rhinol Laryngol 110:729–33, 2001.

21. Belafsky PC, Postma GN, Daniels E, Koufman JA. Transnasal esophagoscopy. Otolaryngol Head Neck Surg;125:588–89, 2001.

22. Belafsky PC, Postma GN, Koufman JA. Laryngopharyngeal reflux symptoms improve before changes in physical findings. Laryngoscope 111:979–81, 2001.

23. Belafsky PC, Postma GN, Koufman JA. The validity and reliability of the reflux finding score (RFS). Laryngoscope 111:1313–17, 2001.

24. Reulbach TR, Belafsky PC, Blalock PD, Koufman JA, Postma GN. Occult laryngeal pathology in a community-based cohort. Otolaryngol Head Neck Surg 124:448–50, 2001.

25. Johnson PE, Koufman JA, Nowak LJ, Belafsky PC, Postma GN. Ambulatory 24-hour double-probe pH monitoring: The importance of manometry. Laryngoscope 111: 1970–75, 2001.

26. Smoak BR, Koufman JA. Effects of gum chewing on pharyngeal and esophageal pH. Ann Otol Rhinol Laryngol 110:1117–19, 2001.

27. Postma GN, Tomek MS, Belafsky PC, Koufman JA. Esophageal motor function in laryngopharyngeal reflux is superior to that of classic gastroesophageal reflux disease. Ann Otol Rhinol Laryngol 110:1114–16, 2001.

28. Axford SE, Sharp S, Ross PE, Pearson JP, Dettmar PW, Panetti M, Koufman JA. Cell biology of laryngeal epithelial defenses in health and disease: Preliminary studies. Ann Otol Rhinol Laryngol 110:1099–1108, 2001.

29. Tasker A, Dettmar PW, Panetti M, Koufman JA, Birchall JP, Pearson, JP. Reflux of gastric juice and glue ear in children. Lancet 359: 493, 2002.

30. Belafsky PC, Postma GN, Koufman JA. Subglottic edema (pseudosulcus) as a manifestation of laryngopharyngeal reflux. Otolaryngol Head Neck Surg 126:649–52, 2002.

31. Belafsky PC, Postma GN, Amin MR, Koufman JA. Symptoms and findings of laryngopharyngeal reflux. Ear Nose Throat J. 81: 10–3, 2002.

32. Koufman JA, Aviv JE, Casiano RR, Shaw GY. Position statement of the American Academy of Otolaryngology—Head and neck surgery on laryngopharyngeal reflux. Otolaryngol Head Neck Surg 127:32–35, 2002.

33. Koufman JA. Laryngopharyngeal reflux is different from classic gastroesophageal reflux disease. Ear Nose Throat J. 81:7–9 2002.

34. Belafsky PC, Halsey WS, Postma GN, Koufman JA. Distal esophageal meat impaction. Ear Nose Throat J. 81:702, 2002.

35. Koufman JA, Belafsky PC, Daniel E, Bach KK, Postma GN. Prevalence of esophagitis in patients with pH-documented laryngopharyngeal reflux. Laryngoscope 112:1606–09, 2002.

36. Belafsky PC, Postma GN, Koufman JA. Hiatal hernia. Ear Nose Throat J. 81:502, 2002.

37. Koufman JA. Laryngopharyngeal reflux 2002: A new paradigm of airway disease. Ear Nose Throat J 81(9 Suppl 2) 2406, 2002.

38. Cohen JT, Bach KK, Postma GN, Koufman JA. Clinical manifestations of laryngopharyngeal reflux. Ear Nose Throat J. 81:14–23, 2002.

39. Belafsky PC, Postma GN, Koufman JA. Validity and reliability of the reflux symptom index (RSI). J Voice 16:274–77, 2002.

40. Postma GN, Bach KK, Belafsky PC, Koufman JA. The role of transnasal esophagoscopy in head and neck surgery. Laryngoscope 112:2242–43, 2002.

41. Postma GN, Johnson LF, Koufman JA. Treatment of laryngopharyngeal reflux. Ear Nose Throat J. 81:24–6, 2002.

42. Belafsky PC, Postma GN, Koufman JA, Bach KK. Candida esophagitis. Ear Nose Throat J. 81:144, 2002.

43. Holland BW, Koufman JA, Postma GN, McGuirt Jr., WF. Laryngopharyngeal reflux and laryngeal web formation in patients with pediatric recurrent respiratory papillomas. Laryngoscope 112:1926–29, 2002.

44. Belafsky PC, Postma GN, Koufman JA. Esophageal inlet patch. Ear Nose Throat J. 81:18, 2002.

45. Postma GN, Belafsky PC, Aviv JE, Koufman JA. Laryngopharyngeal reflux testing. Ear Nose Throat J. 81:14–8, 2002.

46. Johnston N, Bulmer D, Gill GA, Panetti M, Ross PE, Pearson JP, Pignatelli M, Axford A, Dettmar PW, Koufman JA. Cell biology of laryngeal epithelial defenses in health and disease: Further studies. Ann Otol Rhinol Laryngol 112:481–91, 2003.

47. Cohen JT, Postma GN, Enriquez PS, Koufman JA. Barrett's esophagus. Ear Nose Throat J. 82:422, 2003.

48. Enriquez PS, Cohen JT, Postma GN, Koufman JA. Functional abnormalities of the LES found by TNE. Ear Nose Throat J. 82:498–500, 2003.

49. Johnston N, Knight J, Dettmar PW, Lively MO, Koufman JA. Pepsin and carbonic anhydrase isoenzyme III as diagnostic markers for laryngopharyngeal reflux disease. Laryngoscope 114:2129–34, 2004.

50. Westcott CJ, Hopkins MB, Bach KK, Postma, GN, Belafsky, PC, Koufman, JA. Fundoplication for laryngopharyngeal reflux. J American College of Surgeons 199:23–30, 2004.

51. Halum SL, Postma GN, Johnston C, Belafsky PC, Koufman JA. Patients with isolated laryngopharyngeal reflux are not obese. Laryngoscope 115:1042–5, 2005.

52. Halum SL, Butler SG, Koufman JA, Postma GN. Treatment of globus by upper esophageal sphincter injection with botulinum A toxin. ENT J Ear Nose Throat J. 84:74, 2005.

53. Postma GN, Cohen JT, Belafsky PC, Halum SL, Gupta SK, Bach KK, Koufman JA. Transnasal esophagoscopy revisited (over 700 consecutive cases). Laryngoscope 115:321–3, 2005.

54. Knight J, Lively MO, Johnston N, Dettmar PW, Koufman JA. Sensitive pepsin immunoassay for detection of laryngopharyngeal reflux. Laryngoscope 115:1473–8, 2005.

55. Bach KK, Belafsky PC, Wasylik K, Postma GN, Koufman JA. Validity and reliability of the glottal function index. Arch Otolaryngol Head Neck Surg 131:961–4, 2005.

56. Johnston N, Dettmar PW, Lively MO, Postma GN, Belafsky PC, Birchall M, Koufman JA. Effect of pepsin on laryngeal stress protein (Sep70, Sep53, and Hsp70) response: Role in laryngopharyngeal reflux disease. Ann Otol Rhinol Laryngol 115:47–58, 2005.

57. Carrau RL, Khidr A, Gold KF, Crawley JA, Hillson EM, Koufman JA, Pashos CL. Validation of a quality-of-life instrument for laryngopharyngeal reflux. Arch Otolaryngol Head Neck Surg 131:315–20, 2005.

58. Gill GA, Johnston N, Buda A, Pignatelli M, Pearson J, Dettmar PW, Koufman JA. Laryngeal epithelial defenses against laryngopharyngeal reflux (LPR): Investigations of pepsin, carbonic anhydrase III, pepsin, and the inflammatory response. Ann Otol Rhinol Laryngol 114:913–21, 2005.

59. Johnston N, Dettmar PW, Lively MO, Koufman JA. Effect of pepsin on laryngeal stress protein (Sep70, Sep53, and Hsp70)

response: Role in laryngopharyngeal reflux disease. Ann Otol Rhinol Laryngol 115:47–58, 2006.

60. Halum SL, Postma GN, Bates DD, Koufman JA. Incongruence between histologic and endoscopic diagnoses of Barrett's esophagus using transnasal esophagoscopy. Laryngoscope. 116:303–6, 2006.

61. Johnston N, Dettmar PW, Lively MO, Koufman JA. Effect of pepsin on laryngeal stress protein (Sep70, Sep53, and Hsp70) response: Role in laryngopharyngeal reflux disease. Ann Otol Rhinol Laryngol. 115:47–58, 2006.

62. Johnston N, Dettmar PW, Bishwokarma B, Lively MO, Koufman JA. Activity/stability of human pepsin: Implications for reflux attributed laryngeal disease. Laryngoscope. 117:1036–9, 2007.

63. Rees LE, Pazmany L, Gutowska-Owsiak D, Inman CF, Phillips A, Stokes CR, Johnston N, Koufman JA, Postma G, Bailey M, Birchall MA. The mucosal immune response to laryngopharyngeal reflux. Am J Respir Crit Care Med. 177:1187–93, 2008.

64. Birchall MA, Bailey M, Gutowska-Owsiak D, Johnston N, Inman CF, Stokes CR, Postma G, Pazmary L, Koufman JA, Phillips A, Rees LE. Immunologic response of the laryngeal mucosa to extraesophageal reflux. Ann Otol Rhinol Laryngol. 117:891–5, 2008.

65. Amin MR, Postma GN, Setzen M, Koufman JA. Transnasal esophagoscopy: A position statement from the American Bronchoesophagological Association (ABEA). Otolaryngol Head Neck Surg 138:411–13, 2008.

66. Koufman JA, Block C. Differential diagnosis of paradoxical vocal fold movement. American Journal of Speech and Hearing. 17:327–34, 2008.

67. Koufman JA. Perspective on Laryngopharyngeal Reflux: From Silence to Omnipresence. Classics in Voice and Laryngology. Branski R, Sulica L, Eds., Pages 179–266, Plural Publishing, San Diego, 2009.

68. Koufman JA, Johnston N. Potential benefits of pH 8.8 Alkaline Drinking Water as an Adjunct in the Treatment of Reflux Disease. Ann Otol Rhinol Laryngol121:431–34, 2012.

69. Koufman JA. Effect of long-term low-acid diet on Barrett's esophagus. Unpublished data, 2013.

70. Koufman JA, Huang S. A new, inexpensive, and non-invasive saliva test for reflux: Sensitivity and specificity of a rapid pepsin immunoassay. Presented at the Voice Foundation, Philadelphia, 2014. (Submitted for publication)

71. Pavord ID, Chung KF. Management of chronic cough. Lancet 371:1375–84, 2008.

72. Irwin RS. Chronic cough due to gastroesophageal reflux disease: ACCP evidence-based clinical practice guidelines. Chest 129 (1, Suppl):80S–94S, 2006.

73. Pratter MR, Brightling EB, Boulet LP, Irwin RS. An empiric integrated approach to the management of cough: American

College of Chest Physicians evidence-based clinical practice guidelines. Chest 129:222S–231S, 2006.

74. Patterson RN, Johnston BT, MacMahon J, Heaney LG, McGarvey LP. Oesophageal pH monitoring is of limited value in the diagnosis of "reflux-cough." Eur Respir J 24:724–277, 2004.

75. Qadeer MA, Phillips CO, Lopez AR, et al. Proton pump inhibitor therapy for suspected GERD-related chronic laryngitis: a meta-analysis of randomized controlled trials. Am J Gastroenterol 101:2646–54, 2006.

76. Morice AH. The cough hypersensitivity syndrome: a novel paradigm for understanding cough. Lung 188:S87–S90, 2010.

77. Reavis KM, Morris CD, Gopal DV, Hunter JG, Jobe BA. Laryngopharyngeal reflux symptoms better predict the presence of esophageal adenocarcinoma than typical gastroesophageal reflux symptoms. Ann Surg 239:849–56, 2004.

78. Jeyakumar A, Brickman TM, Haben M. Effectiveness of amitriptyline versus cough suppressants in the treatment of chronic cough resulting from postviral vagal neuropathy. Laryngoscope 116:2108–112, 2006.

79. Koufman JA. Laryngoplasty for vocal cord medialization: An alternative to Teflon. Laryngoscope 96:726–31, 1986.

80. Koufman JA. Surgical correction of dysphonia due to bowing of the vocal cords. Annals of Otol Rhinol Laryngol 98:41–45, 1989.

81. El-Serag HB. Time trends of gastroesophageal reflux disease: A systematic review. Clin Gastroenterol Hepatol 5:17–26, 2007.

82. El-Serag H, Becher A, Jones R. Systematic Review: Persistent Reflux Symptoms on Proton Pump Inhibitor Therapy in Primary Care and Community Studies. Alimentary Pharmacology and Therapeutics. Blackwell Publishing, Ltd., pages 1–18, 2010.

83. Altman KW, Stephens RM, Lyttle CS, et al. Changing impact of gastroesophageal reflux in medical and otolaryngology practice. Laryngoscope 115:1145–53, 2005.

84. Pohl H, Welch HG. The role of overdiagnosis and reclassification in the marked increase of esophageal adenocarcinoma incidence. J Natl Cancer Inst 97:142–6, 2005.

85. Lund O, Hasenkam JM, Aagaard MT, Kimose HH. Time-related changes in characteristics of prognostic significance in carcinomas of the oesophagus and cardia. Br J Surg 76:1301, 1989.

86. Conio M, Blanchi S, Lapertosa G, et al. Long-term endoscopic surveillance of patients with Barrett's esophagus. Incidence of dysplasia and adenocarcinoma: A prospective study. Am J Gastroenterol 98:1931–9, 2003.

87. Zahran H, Bailey C, Garbe P et al. Vital Signs: Asthma Prevalence, Disease Characteristics, and Self-Management Education – United States, 2001–2009. MMWR 60:547–52, 2011.

88. Stovold R, Forrest I, Corris P, et al. Pepsin, a biomarker of gastric aspiration in lung allografts. Am J Respir Crit Car Med 175:1298–1303, 2007.

89. Kelly EA, Parakininkas DE, Werlin SL, *et al.* Prevalence of pediatric aspiration-associated extraesophageal reflux disease. JAMA Otolaryngol Head Neck Surg dol.10.1001/jamaoto.2013.4448, Published online August 29, 2013.

# APPENDIX B:
# WHAT ELSE COULD IT BE?

I believe that most patients with non-pulmonary chronic cough have reflux-related and neurogenic cough. I am not a pulmonologist. I don't treat patients with primary lung disease. However, I do treat patients with reactive airway disease secondary to reflux. I also treat patients whose lung disease (e.g., chronic bronchitis, COPD) is due to airway reflux.

The first responsibility of any clinician seeing a chronic cough patient is to rule out life-threatening disease. Since chronic cough is defined as a cough for more than eight weeks,[1] in the absence of fever or other accompanying symptoms, diagnoses such as pneumonia, pulmonary embolus, and cardiac decompensation are unlikely.

There are key elements in the patient's history that must be routinely explored. Does the patient smoke cigarettes? If so, a chest X-ray as well as pulmonary function testing and/or consultation with a pulmonologist are required, and smoking cessation should become a primary part of the initial treatment.

Nevertheless, we routinely rule out primary lung disease with a minimum of the following:

1. Chest X-ray with chest CT scan if there is any abnormality on the X-ray (or any other reason to suspect primary lung disease);
2. PPD (tuberculosis skin test);
3. PFTs (pulmonary function testing)
4. Pulmonary consultation if for any reason lung disease is suspected.

Once primary lung disease has been ruled out, I begin. My list of diagnoses, ranked in order of occurrence, is again shown in table 14. Having covered the first two causes of non-pulmonary chronic cough (reflux-related and neurogenic cough) already, below are brief descriptions and comments about causes 3 through 13.

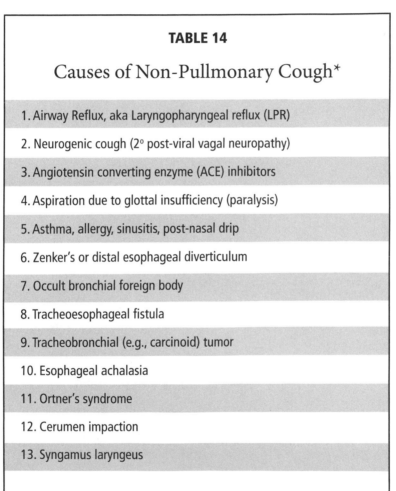

**TABLE 14**

## Causes of Non-Pullmonary Cough*

1. Airway Reflux, aka Laryngopharyngeal reflux (LPR)

2. Neurogenic cough (2° post-viral vagal neuropathy)

3. Angiotensin converting enzyme (ACE) inhibitors

4. Aspiration due to glottal insufficiency (paralysis)

5. Asthma, allergy, sinusitis, post-nasal drip

6. Zenker's or distal esophageal diverticulum

7. Occult bronchial foreign body

8. Tracheoesophageal fistula

9. Tracheobronchial (e.g., carcinoid) tumor

10. Esophageal achalasia

11. Ortner's syndrome

12. Cerumen impaction

13. Syngamus laryngeus

* DISCLOSURE AND DISCLAIMER: This table represents a summary of the author's experience and in no way represents a complete list of all of the possible diagnoses. Furthermore, it is acknowledged that main focus of this book is reflux-related and neurogenic cough, not other (particularly pulmonary) causes of cough.

# Angiotensin Converting Enzyme (ACE) Inhibitors

ACE inhibitors are a class of hypertension (blood pressure) medications associated with chronic cough as a side effect. While some of my chronic cough patients come to me on ACE inhibitors, we manage to change them to an alternative class of medication. By itself, however, ACE inhibitor discontinuance seldom leads to cessation of the chronic cough.

It is possible that ACE inhibitors work by making reflux worse. In any event, for chronic cough patients, this class of medication should be avoided.

# Aspiration Due to Vocal Cord Paralysis (Glottal Insufficiency)

Patients come to me with choking episodes, which may actually represent three different symptoms. First, if food or pills get stuck in the throat or esophagus, it is considered choking. This kind of choking is often related to esophageal reflux. A second type of choking is the inability to get air in. This is usually due to laryngospasm, which in turn is due to airway reflux.

The third type of choking occurs when food or drink goes down the wrong pipe into the trachea and lungs. This is called aspiration, and aspiration can be a complication of vocal cord paralysis. The reason for this is glottal insufficiency; that is, the vocal cords are unable to close properly to prevent aspiration.

Complete closure of the vocal cords during swallowing is an essential function; otherwise, aspiration may lead to pneumonia and even death. If a person coughs every time they drink liquids, this strongly suggests that aspiration is occurring due to vocal cord paralysis. Regardless of cause, any person suspected of having aspiration must be examined by an otolaryngologist.

There are many causes of vocal cord paralysis including viral infections, tumors of the brain, thyroid, neck, and chest, as well as trauma, and neurological diseases. When a patient presents to me with a paralyzed vocal cord, if the cause is not known, I perform a laryngeal examination and laryngeal electromyography. Once the cause of the paralysis is determined, there are specific treatments, including vocal cord surgery, which will correct the problem.[79, 80]

## Asthma, Allergy, Sinusitis, Post-Nasal Drip

The upper airway and the upper digestive tract, the entire aerodigestive system, face a continual assault from the outside world, that is, everything external to the self. These include viruses, bacteria, irritants, and toxins in the air, allergens, and the weather. Thus, the lining membranes of the nose, throat, sinuses, breathing passages, and lungs are all susceptible to many different insults that may have a cumulative effect.

Among the most common symptoms of airway reflux are post-nasal drip, chronic throat clearing, and too much throat mucus. Such symptoms follow a final common pathway, because mucus provides an important mucosal defence.

Mucus is a protective cover for the mucosa (lining membranes) of the nose and throat, but anything that causes inflammation can lead to increased mucus production and its symptoms. We all make about a quart of mucus a day, but with infection, allergy, reflux, and environmental factors (such as winter dryness, mold, and toxic fumes), we make more.

The upper aerodigestive tract is one integrated unit, and allergies, sinusitis, and any infection and irritant will adversely affect the integrity of the lining membranes. Thus, people with allergies and sinusitis will often experience a worsening of their reflux. Conversely, people with airway reflux are more susceptible to infections, viral or otherwise.

Finally, there is a complex, two-way relationship between reflux and true asthma, as there is between true sinusitis and pseudo-sinusitis. Sinusitis or asthma can worsen reflux, and reflux can worsen (true) sinusitis or asthma. Airway reflux does *cause* sinusitis, asthma, and pseudo-asthma and can be an inciting or complicating factor for almost any kind of upper aerodigestive symptom and disease. Conversely, sinusitis and asthma can also worsen reflux.

"Post-nasal drip" is not a diagnosis, and airway reflux and allergies are its most common causes. In other words, post-nasal drip is not a cause of chronic cough.

## Zenker's or Distal Esophageal Diverticulum

Out-pouchings of the esophagus, called diverticula, (singular, diverticulum) can occur as a result of reflux and abnormal esophageal function. A pouch at the upper end of the esophagus is called a *Zenker's diverticulum*; and at the bottom of the esophagus, a *distal esophageal diverticulum*.

Zenker's are far more frequently the cause of symptoms, including bringing up undigested food into the throat (especially when lying down) and chronic cough. Diagnosis is by endoscopy or barium swallow/esophagogram. The bigger the pouch, the more likely it is to cause problems. For pouches larger than four to six centimeters, the treatment is usually surgical removal.

## Occult Bronchial Foreign Body

Both adults and children sometimes have food go down the wrong pipe and wind up in the lung. Sometimes the aspiration event is known, and sometimes it goes unnoticed.

If a piece of food ends up in the lung, it is called a foreign body and can cause chronic cough. This is one of the reasons that I recommend a chest X-ray for all chronic cough patients. It is important to rule out a suspected occult (hidden and unknown) foreign body, which requires removal by bronchoscopy (lung endoscopy).

## Tracheoesophageal Fistula (T-E Fistula)

The *esophagus* (swallowing tube) and the *trachea* (breathing tube) are usually separated by an anatomic common wall so that material that is swallowed cannot get into the airway (trachea). Sometimes there is a hole in that common wall that can be congenital, traumatic, or iatrogenic.

The result is that liquids, and sometimes foods, that are swallowed go into the trachea and lungs, which causes coughing. To diagnose a *tracheoesophageal fistula*, endoscopy and a barium swallow/esophagogram are performed. Treatment is surgery to close the *T-E fistula*.

## Trachebronchial (Carcinoid) Tumor

*Carcinoid tumor* of the trachea is a rare and uncommon cause of cough. It can cause variable degrees of airway obstruction and may be confused with asthma. The presumptive diagnosis is made by pulmonary function testing, and the definitive diagnosis by endoscopy and biopsy. Removal of the tumor resolves the cough.

## Esophageal Achalasia

*Esophageal achalasia* is an *autoimmune esophageal motility disorder* involving the muscular layers of the esophagus and the *lower esophageal sphincter* (LES). It is characterized by failure of the LES to relax and failure of the esophagus to empty.

People with achalasia have difficulty swallowing, chest pain, and chronic cough, as undigested food backs up into the throat. The diagnosis is made by esophageal manometry and barium swallow/esophagography. Treatment is with *Botox* of the LES, *esophageal dilation,* or surgery.

## Ortner's Syndrome

*Ortner's syndrome* is a rare but very interesting cause of chronic cough. The *recurrent laryngeal nerve* descends into the chest where it wraps around the aorta, the large artery coming out of the heart. When a person is in heart failure, the heart literally becomes heavy and can stretch the recurrent laryngeal nerve. This can cause chronic cough as the sensory part of the nerve is part of the vagus. Thus, Ortner's syndrome is the association of chronic cough with congestive heart failure. Ortner's Syndrome can also be a cause of vocal cord paralysis; and aspiration can result (and another potential cause of chronic cough.) When the heart failure is treated, the vocal cord paralysis and chronic cough go away.

## Cerumen Impaction

*Cerumen impaction* is another rare cause of chronic cough. Strange as it sounds, the vagus nerve sends a sensory branch to the ear, specifically to the ear canal. The branch is called Arnold's nerve.

Cerumen, a fancy word for ear wax, when impacted in the ear canal, can stimulate Arnold's nerve and lead to chronic cough. Treatment is simply removal of the impacted ear wax.

## Syngamus Laryngeus

*Syngamus laryngeus* is also rare but can cause chronic cough. Syngamus is gapeworm, a parasitic worm, found in the Caribbean that can be ingested from infected fruit or vegetables. Once ingested the worm can crawl back up into the larynx or trachea. The diagnosis is made by laryngeal examination, and the treatment is endoscopic removal of the worms.

# APPENDIX C: GLOSSARY*

**ACE inhibitor (angiotensin-converting enzyme inhibitor).** ACE inhibitors are a class of hypertension (high-blood pressure) medication believed to cause reflux and chronic cough. The cough related to this medication is probably reflux related.

**Achalasia.** A disease of the esophagus in which its normal motility is lost creating a poorly emptying organ that can become dilated and lead to symptoms of dysphagia (difficulty swallowing) and aspiration. Achalasia is believed to be an autoimmune disorder.

**Acid.** Containing hydrogen ions, pH<7; see *pH scale.* The acidity of stomach acid is pH 1–4, and the same can be said of every fruit and soft drink, with ascorbic, citric, and phosphoric acids being the most commonly used acidic preservatives.

**Acid reflux.** A lay term for symptoms or disease caused by the backflow of gastric (stomach) contents upward into the esophagus (swallowing tube from the throat to the stomach) and airway (sinuses, nose, throat, mouth, breathing passages, and lungs). The most common symptoms of acid reflux are heartburn, indigestion, hoarseness, asthma, post-nasal drip, and cough.

**Acid suppressive, acid suppression.** This refers to decreasing the amount of acid produced by the stomach, specifically reducing the amount of acid produced by the acid-secreting cells.

---

**Acid-suppressive medications**. Acid-suppressive (stomach-acid-reducing) medications generally fall into two classes, proton-pump inhibitors (PPIs) and H2-antagonists (H2As). The PPIs (including Prilosec, Nexium, Dexilant, Prevacid, Protonix, Aciphex) are stronger and associated with frequent side effects and rebound hyperacidity when stopped. The H2As (including Tagamet and Pepcid) have fewer side effects, work better at night, and are generally preferred to PPIs as over-the-counter, taken as needed antireflux medications. See *proton-pump inhibitor* and *H2-antagonist* for more information.

**Aerodigestive tract, aerodigestive**. The airway and digestive tracts treated as one anatomical and functional system. The airway starts at the nose and ends at the root of the lungs; it also includes the throat, larynx (voice box), trachea, bronchial tubes, and lungs. The digestive tract starts at the mouth and ends at the anus; it includes the mouth, throat, esophagus, stomach, and intestines. The airway and digestive tracts comprise one integrated biologic system. See also *integrated aerodigestive medicine*.

**Airway**. The breathing passages, including the nose, sinuses, throat, voice box (larynx), trachea, bronchi, and lungs.

**Airway reflux**. The backflow (reflux) of stomach contents into the airway. Airway reflux is also sometimes called laryngopharyngeal reflux (LPR) or extraesophageal reflux. Airway reflux causes many throat, sinus, and lung diseases and may be confused with other conditions such asthma, allergies, and sinusitis.

**Airway reflux testing**. Reflux testing for the detection of airway reflux; see *pH monitoring*.

**Albuterol**. Albuterol is a medication usually used to treat asthma. It works by dilating (opening) the bronchial tubes; thus it is a bronchodilator-type medication.

**Alkaline**. Not acid, pH>7; see *pH scale*.

**Alkaline water**. Water that has a pH value of more than 7 is technically alkaline; drinking water pH>8 is a useful adjunctive treatment for airway reflux, because pepsin is denatured (dies) at pH>8.

**Allergist**. Doctor who specializes in the diagnosis and treatment of allergies and allergic conditions.

**Allergy**. Abnormal reaction of the body to a previously encountered foreign substance (often animal or plant matter) introduced by inhalation, ingestion, injection, or skin contact, often manifested by itchy eyes, runny nose, nasal congestion, wheezing, skin rash, or diarrhea; a hypersensitivity reaction.

**Ambulatory pH monitoring**. This is an outpatient reflux-testing procedure in which a special, ultra-thin tube is placed through the nose and into the throat and esophagus. The tube is attached to a minicomputer that stores data from pH (acid) sensors embedded in the tube. The pH sensors detect acid in the throat and esophagus. pH monitoring is usually performed for a twenty-four-hour period, and the throat pH sensor provides crucial data and information for the diagnosis of airway (LPR) reflux.

**Ambulatory surgery center (ASC)**. Facility in which day-surgery is performed, with no overnight stay. ASCs are typically used for less serious procedures than those performed in hospital operating rooms. Endoscopic procedures, for example, are often performed in ASCs. In the United States, over 10 million endoscopic procedures a year are performed in ASCs.

**American Beverage Association (ABA).** The ABA represents the beverage industry in the United States, including bottlers of soft drinks, bottled water, and other non-alcoholic beverages. It was founded in 1919 as the American Bottlers of Carbonated Beverages. In 1966, it changed its name to the National Soft Drink Association, and then in 2004 to the ABA. The ABA lobbies for programs supported by its membership.

**Amitriptyline (Elavil).** An old and still commonly prescribed medication in the class of drugs known as tricyclic antidepressants. Interestingly, it is rarely used to treat depression today but usually prescribed for anxiety, tension and migraine headaches, and neurogenic cough. For neurogenic cough, amitriptyline in low doses (5 to 25 mg. before bed) is the single most effective one-drug treatment. When given in small doses at bedtime, side effects such as sleepiness and mouth dryness are uncommon.

**Angiotensin-converting enzyme (ACE) inhibitors.** ACE inhibitors are a class of hypertension (high-blood pressure) medication that causes reflux and chronic cough. It appears that the cough related to this medication is due to reflux.

**Antireflux medication (medical treatment).** Such includes antacids (such as Tums, Rolaids, Gaviscon) as well as H2-antagonists and proton-pump inhibitors.

**Antireflux surgery**. This is a type of surgery used to treat reflux. The most effective and popular procedure is lap fundoplication, in which the dome of the stomach is loosened up and then wrapped around the esophagus and sewed there to create a tight angle so that what goes into the stomach stays in the stomach. This surgery is the best treatment available for reflux; that is, it is better than any medication. Surgery of this type is reserved for special cases since most reflux can be cured by healthy dietary and lifestyle changes.

**Aphonia**. No voice. No contact between the two vocal cords, resulting in no voice, as seen with severe vocal cord paralysis.

**ASC**. See *ambulatory surgery center.*

**Aspiration**. Aspiration occurs when food or liquid is inhaled, spilled, or swallowed into the interior of the voice box and/or into the bronchi and lungs. Laymen refer to this as something "going down the wrong pipe." Aspiration usually causes intense and violent coughing and can lead to pneumonia. Aspiration is one of the symptoms that people call choking.

**Asthma**. Form of reactive airway disease characterized by constriction of the bronchi (the large airway tubes between the lower throat and the lungs); asthma is associated with difficulty getting air out (exhalation) and this type of airway obstruction (only during expiration) is called wheezing.

**Atypical reflux disease**. This is another term (sometimes used by gastroenterologists) for airway reflux, also known as LPR (laryngopharyngeal reflux).

**Autoimmune esophageal motility disorder.** This describes the proposed mechanism for esophageal achalasia in which the smooth muscle of the esophagus is attacked by a person's own white blood cells leading to inflammation, damage, and loss of esophageal function (motility, movement).

**Autonomic, autonomic nerve.** Pertaining to the autonomic nervous system, which controls biologic activities, functions, and behaviors produced by spontaneous internal forces or causes; see below.

**Autonomic nervous system.** The "automatic" nervous system; the system of nerves that innervate (control) blood vessels, heart, smooth muscles (e.g., swallowing), viscera (abdominal organs), and glands. The autonomic nervous system (through autonomic nerves) controls involuntary functions and consists of opposing sympathetic and parasympathetic portions.

**Barium swallow/esophagogram.** This is a video X-ray study of the swallowing mechanism. By swallowing a radio-opaque substance, barium, the entire tube of the throat and esophagus may be seen in real time. The barium swallow is not considered a good diagnostic for reflux; its main use is to examine for structural changes, e.g., cancer, diverticulum.

**Barrett's esophagus.** Refers to abnormal changes in the lining membrane and the cells of the lower portion of the esophagus. When the normal squamous epithelium lining of the esophagus is replaced by gastric (stomachlike) or intestinal columnar epithelium, Barrett's esophagus is diagnosed. The medical significance of Barrett's it that it is considered a precursor to esophageal adenocarcinoma, a particularly lethal cancer. Barrett's is seen in approximately 8–10 percent of refluxers. Once considered irreversible, Barrett's can be reversed by long-term low-acid, low-fat diet.

**Bell's palsy**. A suddenly occurring, facial paralysis that distorts one side of the face. It is believed to be caused by a viral infection of the facial nerve. It is named after Charles Bell (1774–1842), an anatomist, who first described it.

**Botox**. Botox is a popular term for botulinum toxin, a bacteria-derived toxin used in medicine to treat a variety of conditions including voice and swallowing disorders such as spasmodic dysphonia, esophageal achalasia, and Zenker's diverticulum. Botox is most widely known for its use in the treatment of facial wrinkles.

**Bronchial, bronchus, bronchi**. Referring to the bronchi, which are the two main breathing tubes and their branch points inside the lungs.

**Bronchodilators**. Type of medicine used to open up the bronchi when they are narrowed during an asthma attack or for other reactive airways disorders.

**Bronchoscopy**. Endoscopy (internal examination) of the lungs, usually performed by a pulmonologist or otolaryngologist.

**Candida (fungal) esophagitis**. Candida is a commonly occurring fungus that is associated with disease in many areas of the body, including the mouth, throat, and esophagus. Candida esophagitis is often reflux related. It is believed that reflux alters the normal bacterial flora of the esophagus to allow the fungus to thrive. Candida esophagitis is treated with orally administered anti-fungal drugs. A more serious, ulcerative, sometimes life-threatening variation of Candida esophagitis is sometimes seen in patients with AIDS.

**Carcinoid tumor**. A relatively uncommon tumor that grows in the trachea or bronchi, the presentation of which may be confused with asthma. It is an uncommon cause of chronic cough

**CCI**. See *chronic cough index*.

**Cerumen, cerumen impaction**. Cerumen is ear wax and a cerumen impaction means that the ear canal is blocked up by wax that is tightly packed. Cerumen impaction can be a cause of chronic chough mediated by a branch of the vagus that goes to the ear, Arnold's nerve.

**Choking, choking episodes**. There are three different symptoms that people call choking: 1. if food or pills get stuck in the throat or esophagus, the choking is often related to narrowing of the esophagus due to esophageal reflux; 2. inability to get air in during inhalation, usually due to laryngospasm, which is also usually caused by airway reflux; finally, 3. choking occurs when food or drink "goes down the wrong pipe" into the trachea and lungs. This is called aspiration, and it can be a complication of vocal cord paralysis or glottal insufficiency,

**Chronic bronchitis**. Bronchitis is one of the most common causes of chronic cough and results from inflammation and infection in the airways of the lung. Bronchitis may be due to viral, bacterial, or fungal infection and it may be a consequence of airway reflux. Cigarette smoking may also cause chronic bronchitis.

**Chronic cough.** Defined as cough lasting more than eight weeks.

**Chronic cough index (CCI).** A symptom index invented by this book's author, Dr. Jamie Koufman, to help diagnose and differentiate reflux-related from neurogenic chronic cough.

**Chronic obstructive lung disease (COPD).** This is a mixed-bag diagnosis that includes chronic bronchitis, bronchiectasis, and emphysema. Is it usually caused by smoking, airway reflux, infection, and/or exposure to environmental contaminants or toxins.

**Cimetidine (Tagamet).** Introduced in 1979, cimetidine was the first really effective acid-suppressive medication. It is an H2-antagonist, and it is still considered to be a safe and effective antireflux medication.

**Columnar (gastric) epithelium.** This is the normal lining mucosa (membrane) of the stomach and intestines; it is seen in Barrett's esophagus when it grows up into the esophagus.

**Contact Ulcer.** This is a condition of the larynx in which the cartilage of the arytenoid becomes exposed, causing throat pain and pain referred to the ear. It is caused most commonly by airway reflux and from intubation for ventilation during general anesthesia.

**COPD.** See *chronic obstructive lung disease.*

**Cough hypersensitivity syndrome.** This is an outdated, non-specific, diagnostic term that some physicians use to describe neurogenic and reflux-related cough. Use of this general term implies that a specific cause or diagnosis has not been identified.

**Diaphragm**. A flat, bellows-like muscle that separates the abdominal cavity from the chest cavity and is vital for respiration.

**Diffuse polyneuropathy**. A neuropathy that involves several nerves as seen in post-viral vagal neuropathy.

**Digestive tract**. All parts of the body involved in eating, swallowing, and digesting nutrients, including the mouth, tongue, throat, esophagus, duodenum, liver, pancreas, small intestine (jejunum and ileum), large bowel (colon), rectum, and anus.

**Distal esophageal diverticulum**. An outpouching of the lower esophagus that can trap undigested food and cause dysphagia (difficulty swallowing and chronic cough), usually seen in elderly patients.

**Duodenum**. Uppermost part of the small intestine that connects the stomach to the small bowel (jejunum); the gall bladder and pancreas drain into the duodenum.

**Dysfunction**. Malfunctioning, as of an organ or structure of the body; "bad function."

**Dysphagia**. Difficulty swallowing.

**Dysphonia**. Hoarseness, "bad voice."

**EGD**. See *esophagogastroduodenoscopy*.

**Elavil**. See *amitriptyline*.

**Empiric treatment**. Initiation of treatment prior to determination of a firm diagnosis with the implication that the diagnosis is uncertain and positive response to treatment may be considered as diagnostic.

**Endoscope, endoscopy**. An instrument (or procedure) used to examine a hollow organ such as the esophagus. Endoscopic examination of the esophagus with an esophagoscope is called esophagoscopy. Examination of the lungs, bronchoscopy, using a bronchoscope and examination of the colon, colonoscopy, using a colonoscope are other examples of endoscopy and endoscopes.

**Enigma, enigmatic**. A puzzling or inexplicable occurrence or situation; or a person of puzzling, incongruous, or inexplicable nature.

**Enigmatic chronic cough**. A puzzling, inexplicable, and undiagnosed chronic (more than eight weeks duration) cough. Most people who fall into this group have seen many doctors and had many ineffective treatments.

**ENT (ear, nose, and throat) physician**. Medical specialist in diseases of the ears, nose, and throat; the specialty is called otorhinolaryngology or otolaryngology—head and neck surgery.

**Erosive esophagitis**. Reflux-related esophageal damage causing ulceration to the lining membrane (mucosa) in the area above the stomach. This diagnosis requires esophagoscopy and biopsy and is a complication of esophageal reflux, aka GERD, gastroesophageal reflux disease.

**Esophageal achalasia.** An idiopathic (probably autoimmune) condition that affects esophageal motility (movement) by damaging its smooth muscle layer. In achalasia, the lower esophageal sphincter (valve) also fails to relax, and the esophagus can become distended leading to dysphagia (swallowing difficulties), regurgitation, aspiration, and cough.

**Esophageal cancer.** The prevalence of esophageal cancer has grown 850 percent since the 1970s, and it is the fastest growing cancer in the United States. Most esophageal cancer is caused by reflux. These are called adenocarcinomas, and they generally occur in the area where the esophagus meets the stomach. When detected, most cases of esophageal cancer are advanced and deadly, so that early detection is an important goal. Transnasal esophagoscopy is indicated for people who have long-standing reflux, and its airway reflux, not just people with esophageal reflux (GERD). Indeed, some studies have shown that chronic cough is the symptom most often associated with the development of esophageal cancer.

**Esophageal dilation.** To dilate is to stretch from the inside; esophageal dilation is stretching of the esophagus using dilators or bougies, usually introduced through the mouth during endoscopy.

**Esophageal erosions.** Complication of gastroesophageal reflux disease in which there is breakdown of the esophageal lining (mucosa), ulceration.

**Esophageal reflux.** Backflow of gastric (stomach) contents into the esophagus.

**Esophageal spasm**. One of the mechanisms for reflux-caused chest pain, even crushing chest pain that can mimic a heart attack.

**Esophageal stricture**. With prolonged chronic or chronic intermittent gastroesophageal reflux disease, the esophagus can become scarred and narrowed, leading to dysphagia and food sticking in the stricture. These scarred narrowings can be stretched open by esophageal dilation, but stricture formation is a sign that reflux treatment should be escalated.

**Esophageal varices**. Varices are extremely dilated veins in the wall of the esophagus, and they are usually associated with severe liver damage (cirrhosis).

**Esophagitis**. Inflammation of the esophagus, associated with reflux disease; biopsies will show many inflammatory cells.

**Esophagogastroduodenoscopy (EGD)**. Examination of the esophagus, stomach, and duodenum (upper small bowel) usually performed by a gastroenterologist under sedation. EGD is not the best way to examine the esophagus in reflux patients; unsedated transnasal esophagoscopy is preferred because it is a safer, more accurate, and less expensive examination.

**Esophagus**. The muscular swallowing tube that connects the throat and the stomach; the esophagus has two valves, one at the top where it attaches to the pharynx (throat) and one at the bottom where it attaches to the stomach. The top and bottom esophageal valves are called the upper esophageal sphincter (UES) and the lower esophageal sphincter (LES).

**Expiratory**. Of or relating to exhalation, breathing out.

**Expiratory wheezing**. Noisy breathing on exhalation characterized by restricted and prolonged exhalation, usually due to asthma.

**Extraesophageal reflux disease**. Reflux that comes up above the esophagus into the throat; synonym for airway reflux and laryngopharyngeal reflux.

**Facility fee**. The amount of money charged and collected by a medical facility, such as an ambulatory surgery center, for use of the facility. The facility fee is independent of (over and above) professional fees, e.g., for endoscopy, EGD.

**Famotidine (Pepcid)**. This acid-suppressive medication is an H2-antagonist. It is a safe and effective over-the-counter, antireflux medication suitable for use without a doctor's prescription. It is similar to cimetidine.

**Food and Drug Administrations (FDA)**. Branch of government responsible for monitoring drug and food quality and safety. The GRAS (generally regarded as safe) list is approved by the FDA. In 1973, the FDA decided that acid would be the main preservative for foods and beverages in bottles and cans, and acids make up 13 percent of the GRAS food additive list.

**Fundoplication, laparoscopic fundoplication**. Antireflux surgical procedure performed by freeing the dome (fundus) of the stomach and sewing (plicating) it around the esophagus to create a tight angle so that food in the stomach stays in the stomach; that is, prevents reflux. Laparoscopic means that the surgery is done with small instruments used through very small openings, meaning, there is no abdominal incision needed for this approach.

**Fundus.** Dome or upper portion of the stomach. When a person has antireflux surgery, the dome of the stomach, the fundus, is loosed and then wrapped and sewed around the esophagus.

**Gabapentin (Neurontin).** Originally developed for treatment of epilepsy but hardly ever used for that purpose. It is primarily used for the treatment of neurogenic pain such as in diabetics with neuropathic foot pain and for fibromyalgia. Gabapentin appears to improve vagal function and is particularly successful in treating post-viral vagal neuropathy and symptoms such as chronic sore throat, burning tongue, odynophonia (painful speaking) and neurogenic cough. Gabapentin comes in a variety of doses that make it easily titrated (customized) for each patient's needs.

**Gastric.** Of or relating to the stomach.

**Gastroenterologist (GI).** An internal medicine specialist physician whose focus is the gastrointestinal (digestive) tract.

**Gastroesophageal reflux disease (GERD).** This is the most commonly used medical term for esophageal reflux. Literally it means "stomach-esophagus backflow disease."

**Gastroparesis.** Paresis means "partial paralysis." Gastroparesis is partial paralysis of the stomach, and in lay terms, this condition is sometimes called "lazy stomach." Gastroparesis is associated with symptoms of nausea, bloating, and abdominal discomfort or pain. Gastroparesis may be caused by post-viral vagal neuropathy, and it is usually treated with medications to improve the motility (movement) of the gastrointestinal tract.

**GI**. See *gastroenterologist*.

**Globus, globus pharyngeus**. A sensation of a lump in the throat, a common symptom of airway reflux; usually caused by UES (upper esophageal sphincter) dysfunction.

**Glottal closure index (GCI)**. A symptom index created by the author of this book, Dr. Jamie Koufman, to assess the degree of voice impairment caused by glottal closure problems such as vocal cord paralysis and paresis (partial paralysis).

**Glottal closure symptoms**. Symptoms may include: voice change, labored speaking, painful speaking, vocal fatigue (voice worsens with prolonged use), breathiness and air wasting, and diplophonia (double tone). See also *glottal closure index*.

**Glottal insufficiency**. General term for condition of the larynx and vocal cords resulting from a glottal closure problem; term applied to aphonia and/or dysphonia associated with vocal cord paralysis and paresis; air wasting and aspiration may result.

**Granuloma**. This is a benign growth that occurs in the larynx; associated with trauma (e.g. endotracheal intubation) and airway reflux.

**H2A**. See H2-antagonist below.

**H2-antagonist (H2A).** H2As are a class of acid-suppressive medications that are used to treat reflux. H2As are safe and do not need to be administered by a physician; they do not cause rebound hyperacidity and may be used on an as-needed basis. Most common medications are:

| GENERIC NAME | TRADE NAME |
|---|---|
| cimetidine | Tagamet |
| famotidine | Pepcid |

**Heartburn.** Chest pain related to reflux, usually after a large or fatty meal. It may be sometimes confused with a heart attack.

**Hiatal hernia.** An anatomic slippage of the lower esophageal sphincter above the diaphragm. By itself, a hiatal hernia is no a reason for antireflux surgery.

**High-definition airway and esophageal ISFET pH monitoring.** New state-of-the-art reflux-testing method invented by the author of this book, Dr. Jamie Koufman. This technology is highly sensitive and specific for diagnosing airway reflux and reflux-related chronic cough. The ISFET chip, usually reserved for use in high-quality pH meters, has greatly increased the accuracy of pH testing for airway reflux.

**Hoarseness.** Abnormal voice, dysphonia, often characterized by roughness and raspiness of the voice.

**Hypopharynx.** The lower part of the throat (pharynx); this includes the larynx (voice box), the piriform sinuses, and the esophageal inlet, which form the uppermost opening into the esophagus.

**Iatrogenic**. Doctor-caused, as in the iatrogenic vocal cord paralysis following thyroid cancer surgery.

**Idiopathic**. Of unknown cause.

**Idiopathic pulmonary fibrosis**. Progressive, chronic lung disease characterized by scarring in the lungs. This condition may be wholly or in part a complication of long-standing airway reflux.

**Idiosyncratic foods**. Idiosyncratic means something peculiar to an individual. Idiosyncratic foods are foods that cause reflux in some people but not in others; an individual's trigger foods for reflux. Among the most common idiosyncratic foods (across the population) are onions, garlic, tomatoes, nuts, wine, coffee, and chocolate.

**Indigestion**. Discomfort or difficulty digesting food, also called dyspepsia, may be associated with burping (eructation), gas, and heartburn.

**Induction (detox) reflux diet**. Dr. Koufman's strict, two-week diet—low-fat, low-acid, no alcohol, no eating within four hours of bed—is phase one for people with airway and esophageal reflux.

**Inspiratory**. Of or relating to inhalation, breathing in. Inspiratory stridor, for example, refers to noisy breathing during inhalation.

**Inspiratory stridor**. Noisy breathing on inspiration. Stridor means noisy breathing.

**Integrated aerodigestive medicine (IAM)**. This is a new term for a new field, coined by the author of this book, Dr. Jamie Koufman, which encompasses parts of otolaryngology, gastroenterology, and pulmonology. Crossing traditional medical specialty lines, this new specialty focuses on all symptoms and diseases of the aerodigestive tract and the vagus nerve.

**ISFET**. ISFET is a chip (device) used to measure pH (acidity) in top-quality pH meters and diagnostic pH-monitoring systems. ISFET stands for "ion-sensitive field-effect transistor." For airway reflux testing, ISFET is superior to older technology.

**Laparoscopic (lap) fundoplication**. Antireflux surgical procedure performed by freeing up the dome (fundus) of the stomach and sewing (plicating) it around the esophagus to create a tight angle so that food in the stomach stays in the stomach; that is, prevents reflux. Laparoscopic refers to performing the fundoplication operation though multiple mini-incisions. (As of this writing, laparoscopic fundoplication is still the best surgical reflux treatment available.)

**Laryngeal electromyography (LEMG)**. A neuro-diagnostic test in which a laryngologist places small needle electrodes into muscles of the larynx to evaluate the superior and recurrent laryngeal nerves; this test is used to evaluate vocal cord paresis and to make the diagnosis of post-viral-vagal neuropathy.

**Laryngeal nerves**. The laryngeal (voice box) nerves that account for voice, cough, and airway protection during swallowing. The main vocal cold nerve is the recurrent laryngeal nerve and a second nerve, the superior laryngeal nerve, allows high-pitched voicing. All of these vocal cord (laryngeal) nerves are branches of the vagus nerve.

**Laryngologist.** A physician, usually an otolaryngologist (ENT doctor), who specializes in problems of the voice and throat, including airway (LPR) reflux.

**Laryngoscopy.** Examination of the larynx (voice box) using a special endoscope designed for that purpose. Today, most laryngoscopies are performed by laryngologists using transnasal high-definition, distal-chip camera and video-recording instrumentation.

**Laryngopharyngeal reflux (LPR).** Former name for airway reflux; LPR is still the most common term in the medical literature for the backflow of stomach contents into the throat. (The author, Dr. Jamie Koufman, coined both terms, *LPR* and *airway reflux.*)

**Laryngospasm.** Laryngospasm is a frightening type of choking episode in which the vocal cords clamp shut causing severe inspiratory stridor. The most common cause of laryngospasm is airway reflux.

**Larynx, laryngeal (voice box).** Housing of the vocal cords, false vocal cords, and the epiglottis (cover). The larynx is responsible for three functions: phonation (voice), airway (it is through the larynx that air gets into the lungs), and sphincteric protection of the airway with swallowing. The sphincteric function of the larynx prevents aspiration by keeping foods or liquids out of the lungs.

**LEMG.** See *laryngeal electromyography.*

**Leukoplakia.** Literally means "white plaque," and when it is present in the voice box (specifically on the vocal cords) it is considered a pre-cancer and should be biopsied.

**Lifestyle factors**. Time of eating, use of tobacco, too-tight belts or clothing, overconsumption of alcohol are all considered to be lifestyle factors that influence reflux. Of all the lifestyle factors, late (night) eating is the most commonly identified problem.

**Longevity phase (fourth phase)**. This final phase of the reflux diet is achieved when a person can live effortlessly maintaining a low-fat, low-acid, pH-balanced diet.

**Lower esophageal sphincter (LES)**. The valve at the lower end of the esophagus where it joins the stomach. The LES opens to let food into the stomach and (in health) prevents esophageal reflux. The antireflux surgical procedure, laparoscopic fundoplication, tightens the LES.

**LPR symptoms**. LPR, laryngopharyngeal reflux, is a synonym for airway reflux. LPR symptoms include hoarseness, chronic throat-clearing and cough, a lump-in-the-throat sensation, too much throat mucus, post-nasal drip, difficulty swallowing, choking episodes, shortness of breath, and asthma.

**Maintenance phase (third phase)**. This is the third phase of the reflux diet when daily and weekly meal plans allow for continuous low-fat, low-acid, pH-balanced eating.

**Motor nerve**. An efferent, travelling from the brain, nerve that conveys impulses that cause muscular contraction.

**Nasopharynx**. The part of the upper throat behind the nose and above the palate.

**Neural plasticity**. Refers to the observation that neural pathways (especially in the brain) can change over time; that nerves can reestablish new connections. The vagus nerve has neural plasticity that can result in spontaneous recovery after PVVN.

**Neurogenic, neuropathic, neurogenic pain**. Of or relating to a nerve; pain that is caused by a neuropathy or malfunctioning nerve.

**Neurogenic cough**. Nerve-caused cough; cough caused by vagal neuropathy, often associated with post-viral vagal neuropathy.

**Neurologist**. An internal medicine specialist physician who specializes in disorders and diseases of the brain and nervous system. Some neurologists perform electromyography, though rarely laryngeal electromyography.

**Neurontin**. See *gabapentin*.

**Neuropathy**. Sick nerve syndrome. Neuropathies may be caused by infections, such as post-viral vagal neuropathy, and by many other causes including trauma (injuries), autoimmune diseases, toxic exposures, and diseases such as diabetes, Lyme's, and MS (multiple sclerosis). Bell's palsy and post-viral vagal neuropathy are common neuropathies.

**Non-pulmonary**. Not of the lung(s), as in non-pulmonary chronic cough. Non-pulmonary implies that a problem in the lungs is *not* the cause of the chronic cough.

**Odynophagia**. Painful swallowing; and may be a sign of reflux, neuropathy, or throat cancer.

**Odynophonia**. Painful speaking, usually a neurogenic symptom, often associated with post-viral vagal neuropathy.

**Otorhinolaryngology, otolaryngology (ORL)**. An ENT (ear, nose, and throat) physician and surgeon who specializes in diseases of the ears, nose, and throat; the specialty is also called otolaryngology—head and neck surgery.

**Oropharynx**. That part of the throat behind the tongue and below the palate. The tonsils and the uvula are in the oropharynx.

**Ortner's syndrome**. Unusual cause of left vocal cord paralysis; syndrome in which an enlarged heart (often in heart failure) stretches the recurrent laryngeal nerve (that wraps around the aorta) leading to left vocal cord paralysis. It is a rare cause of chronic cough.

**Otolaryngologist, otolaryngology**. An ENT (ear, nose and throat) physician and surgeon who specializes in diseases of the ears, nose, and throat; the specialty is also called otolaryngology—head and neck surgery.

**Outcomes instrument**. This refers to a standardized questionnaire used in medical research that allows clinicians to determine if a specific therapy is effective. Validated outcomes instruments have already been proven to be statistically accurate.

**Pachydermia laryngitis**. Archaic term for thickening of the laryngeal lining due to inflammation, particularly of the posterior (back of) the larynx, usually due to airway reflux.

**Paradoxical vocal cord movement (PVCM).** Reversal of the normal phasic movement of the vocal cords with respiration. Under normal circumstances, the vocal cords open slightly during inhalation and close slightly during exhalation. With PVCM, the vocal cords close during inhalation leading to varying degrees of airway obstruction; associated with inspiratory stridor; also, sometimes called VCD (vocal cord dysfunction), another archaic term.

**Paralysis.** Paralysis of a muscle or muscle group occurs when the nerve going to those muscle(s) is interrupted. The most common causes of vocal cord paralysis are viral infections, idiopathic (of unknown cause), post-viral vagal neuropathy, and iatrogenic (doctor-caused), e.g., thyroid cancer surgery.

**Paresis, paretic** (see also *vocal cord paresis*). Partial paralysis, often as a consequence of viral infection, neck trauma, or surgery.

**Paroxysmal laryngospasm.** Acute and severe reversal of the normal phasic movement of the vocal cords. With laryngospasm, the vocal cords close tightly leading to airway obstruction and inspiratory stridor, almost a crowing sound. Typically, patients refer to laryngospasm as terrifying "choking episodes"; these laryngospasm attacks typically last minutes and are almost always caused by airway reflux. See also *laryngospasm*.

**Pepsin.** The primary digestive enzyme of the stomach. Pepsin (and not acid) causes reflux-related tissue damage; it has also been implicated in causing esophageal and laryngeal cancer. (The author now has a non-invasive diagnostic test for reflux that detects pepsin in saliva.)

**Pepsin assay**. A test used to detect or measure pepsin.

**pH, pH scale**. The pH scale takes its name from the words "potential of hydrogen." The pH scale is used to measure the acidity or alkalinity of a substance or solution. The pH scale ranges from 0 to 14, with pH7 being neutral. Numbers above 7 indicate alkalinity and numbers below 7 indicate acidity. The scale is logarithmic, meaning that pH2 is ten times more acidic than pH 3 and one hundred times more acidic than pH4. Stomach acid is typically pH1–4, as are virtually all soft drinks today. Clinically, we know that consumption of beverages pH<4 is associated with reflux disease, particularly with silent airway reflux.

**pH balancing**. pH balancing is a way to reduce the impact of acidic foods by combining them with alkaline, as in having strawberries with low-fat milk (cow, almond, or soy) or with alkaline water.

**pH monitoring**. Reflux-testing method in which an ultra-thin device is swallowed and measures the pH in the throat and esophagus during a twenty-four-hour period. When a pH sensor is placed in the throat, this technology using an ISFET chip is the state of the art for accurately diagnosing airway reflux.

**Pharynx**. The entire throat, from the back of the nose down to the lower end where it joins the esophagus. The uppermost portion is called the nasopharynx and the lower portion is called the laryngopharynx or hypopharynx.

**Pharyngeal**. Of or relating to the pharynx (throat).

**Pharyngeal/UES/esophageal manometry**. A specialized technology that is used to measure the pressures of the throat and esophagus, specifically to assess esophageal function, coordination of the swallowing mechanism, and upper and lower esophageal valve pressures. Manometry is performed by having the patient swallow a thin instrument, introduced through the nose. Manometry takes only about ten minutes to perform; and it is done as part of the reflux testing battery because manometry also determines where to accurately locate the pH sensors for pH monitoring.

**Pleurisy**. Inflammation of the pleura, the outer lining of the lungs, usually caused by a viral infection and characterized by a dry cough and pain, particularly when taking a deep breath.

**Polyneuropathy**. A neuropathic condition involving several nerves, e.g., PVVN.

**Polypoid degeneration**. Also sometimes called Reinke's edema. Excessive floppy swelling of the vocal cords that produces a rough, low-pitched voice; associated with long-term reflux and/or smoking as well as with vocal cord paresis. When necessary, treatment is usually office-based surgical laser removal.

**Post-nasal drip**. The feeling that mucus is dripping into the throat from the back of the nose, and may be due to allergy, infection, toxic fumes, or reflux. Indeed, it is one of the commonest symptoms of airway reflux.

**Post-viral vagal neuropathy (PVVN)**. Viral infections can infect the vagi (plural of vagus) leading to vagal system dysfunction that may involve any of the vagal nerve branches. PVVN, for example, often causes sudden and simultaneous vocal cord paresis and airway reflux. PVVN is a common cause of reflux-related and neurogenic chronic cough. The diagnosis of PVVN may be presumed by the findings on laryngeal examination; however, diagnostic confirmation requires laryngeal electromyography.

**PPI**. See *proton-pump inhibitor.*

**Prokinetic, prokinetic agent**. A class of medications that are "for movement"; usually used to treat esophageal dysmotility and poor esophageal valve function. Contemporary prokinetic agents include reglan, domperidone, erythromycin, and gabapentin.

**Proton-pump inhibitor (PPI)**. A class of acid-suppressive medications used to treat reflux. PPIs should be administered by a physician because they cause rebound hyperacidity when stopped abruptly; and they should not be used on an as-needed basis. In addition, they should not be used long term as they mask progression of disease, leading to complications of reflux including esophageal cancer and pre-cancer, lung, and sinus disease. The most common medications are listed here:

| GENERIC NAME | TRADE NAME |
| --- | --- |
| omeprazole | Prilosec |
| lansoprazole | Prevacid |
| pantaprazole | Protonix |
| esomeprazole | Nexium |
| rabeprazole | Aciphex |

**Pseudo-asthma, pseudo-asthmatics**. A misdiagnosis of asthma. A condition, usually reactive airway disease caused by airway reflux, that is confused with asthma. People with pseudo-asthma, pseudo-asthmatics, usually have inspiratory stridor and not expiratory wheezing.

**Psychogenic cough**. Having origin in the mind or in a mental condition or process; a psychogenic disorder is different from an organic disorder. Psychogenic cough implies that a psychiatric or psychological problem is the cause of the cough. This diagnosis is almost never correct.

**Pulmonary**. Of or relating to the lungs.

**Pulmonary function tests (PFTs)**. A set of breathing tests designed to measure lung volumes and lung function; PFTs are useful in diagnosing reactive airway disease, asthma, and COPD.

**Pulmonologist (PUL)**. Chest physician, a medical doctor who specializes in problems of the lungs.

**PVVN**. *See post-viral vagal neuropathy.*

**Reactive airway disease, reactive airways**. There are many different manifestations and diagnoses associated with the term reactive airways. In all cases, something triggers the airway to change its physiology (usually) in a way that produces altered breathing and distressing symptoms.

**Recalcitrant**. Refractory; resisting control; hard to deal with or manage.

**Recurrent laryngeal nerve**. The main branch of the vagus nerve that controls the vocal cords and voice.

**Reflux**. Backflow; from the Latin: *re*, "back" and *fluere*, "to flow."

**Reflux diet**. A diet designed to improve reflux. The author's reflux diet includes both a strict, short-term (two-week) induction (detox) diet and a long-term diet. Both are low-acid, low-fat diets. For more about this topic, see *Dropping Acid: The Reflux Diet Cookbook & Cure*.

**Reflux esophagitis, esophagitis**. Inflammation of the esophagus, associated with reflux disease; biopsies will show many inflammatory cells.

**Reflux-finding score (RFS)**. The RFS is a validated outcomes instrument for quantifying the laryngeal findings of airway reflux.

**Reflux laryngitis**. See *laryngopharyngeal reflux* and *airway reflux*.

**Reflux symptom index (RSI)**. The RSI is a validated outcomes instrument for quantifying the laryngeal symptoms of airway reflux; take the quiz on page 13.

**Reflux-related cough**. Cough caused by airway reflux.

**Reflux-related reactive airway disease, reactive airway disease**. Most reactive airway disease, with the exception of allergic rhinitis, is due to airway reflux; see also *laryngospasm*.

**Reflux testing**. A diagnostic method for documenting abnormal reflux in the airway and esophagus; the state of the art is high-definition airway and esophageal ISFET pH monitoring.

**Reflux-to-neurogenic (R:N) ratio**. This tool devised by Dr. Koufman is a useful diagnostic. The R:N ratio is determined by adding up the answers to the ten questions in the two columns in the chronic cough index. The R:N ratio will suggest a likely diagnosis. When the R:N ratio is 10:0, 9:1, or 8:2, the presumptive diagnosis is reflux-related cough. When the R:N ratio is 2:8, 1:9, or 0:10, the presumptive diagnosis is neurogenic cough. When the R:N ratio is 7:3, 6:4, 5:5, 4:6, or 3:7, the likely diagnosis is both reflux-related and neurogenic cough.

**Refluxate**. A term for the actual material that refluxes; that is, it is the liquid mixture (composed of acid, stomach enzymes, and undigested food) that comes up.

**Refractory**. Hard or impossible to manage; resisting ordinary methods of treatment.

**Regurgitation**. The backflow of material from the esophagus or stomach into the mouth. People with regurgitation also may complain of heartburn, indigestion, and a sour taste in the mouth.

**Respiratory reflux**. Respiratory reflux is a synonym for LPR or airway reflux. The new term is more intuitive. It is obviously reflux into the respiratory tract.

**Reinke's edema (aka polypoid degeneration)**. Excessive floppy swelling of the vocal cords that produces a rough low-pitched voice; associated with long-term reflux, hypothyroidism, and smoking, as well as with vocal cord paresis.

**RFS**. See *reflux-finding score*.

**RSI**. See *reflux symptom index.*

**Sensory, sensory nerve**. Pertaining to the senses or sensation, or a nerve that passes impulses from receptors toward or to the central nervous system (the brain), an afferent nerve.

**Silent airway reflux**. This is an important compound term, which connects airway reflux (LPR) with silent reflux; that is, airway reflux that occurs without obvious esophageal reflux symptoms of heartburn and indigestion.

**Silent reflux**. Silent reflux is reflux that occurs without the obvious symptoms of heartburn and indigestion. Within the context of this book, the term *silent reflux* is usually synonymous with silent airway reflux. But theoretically, silent airway reflux is differentiated from silent esophageal reflux. Even esophageal reflux sometimes can be silent; that is, occurring without typical esophageal symptoms.

·**Sinusitis**. Inflammation and/or infection of the sinuses that may be caused by upper-respiratory infection, allergy, or airway reflux.

**Sleep apnea**. A condition in which a person stops breathing during sleep; most cases are due to obesity, abnormal throat anatomy, and/or airway reflux. Snoring and generally noisy breathing are typical as well as daytime somnolence (sleepiness).

**Spontaneous activity**. This finding of random electrical activity seen on laryngeal electromyography suggests ongoing neural denervation (nerve damage). Such is usually associated with a pathologic process that involves the affected nerve(s).

**Squamous epithelium**. The normal lining mucosa (membrane) of the esophagus.

**Stridor**. Noisy (audible) breathing. Stridor may be inspiratory, expiratory, or both. Inspiratory stridor is associated with reflux and expiratory stridor (wheezing) is associated with asthma.

**Stroboscopy, videostroboscopy**. An exam used by laryngologists for studying the motion of the vocal cords, especially the vocal cord vibrations, by making the motion appear to slow down by periodically illuminating the vocal cords. Usually, stroboscopy is recorded on a video system for slow-motion playback and analysis. It can show vocal cord stiffness, scarring, or weakness (paresis).

**Superior laryngeal nerve**. A small branch of the vagus nerve that controls the tension of the vocal cords and high pitch of the voice.

**Supraesophageal reflux disease**. This is a synonym for laryngopharyngeal reflux and airway reflux.

**Syngamus laryngeus**. A parasitic worm indigenous to the Caribbean, which once ingested can reside in the larynx just below the vocal cords; it is a rare cause of chronic cough.

**Tagamet (cimetidine)**. Acid-suppressive medication; see *cimetidine*.

**TB**. See *tuberculosis*.

**T-E (tracheoesophageal) fistula**. An anatomic defect or opening in the common wall that separates the esophagus from the trachea.

Such an opening (fistula) leads to aspiration; that is, food and drink that is swallowed goes into the lungs. T-E fistulas may be congenital, traumatic, or iatrogenic, and they usually require surgical closure (repair).

**TFL**. See *transnasal flexible laryngoscopy*.

**Therapeutic trial**. Deductive use of a specific treatment to make a specific diagnosis; that is, empiric treatment used as a diagnostic. If a treatment effectively alleviates a certain condition, it is assumed that the condition was the correct diagnosis.

**Throatburn**. Throatburn is a symptom like heartburn, which may be related to airway reflux or vagal neuropathy, e.g., post-viral vagal neuropathy. Indeed, the cause of throatburn is usually neurogenic.

**Trachea**. The main breathing tube that connects the bottom of the larynx (voice box) with the bronchi and lungs.

**Trachebronchial**. Of or relating to the trachea and bronchial tubes.

**Trachebronchial tumor**. Benign or malignant tumor in the large airway, either trachea or bronchi.

**Tracheoesophageal fistula (TE fistula)**. An opening between the esophagus and the trachea that causes aspiration, contamination of the airway, by whatever is swallowed, including saliva. The origin of a TE fistula may be congenital, traumatic, or iatrogenic.

**Tramadol (Ultram)**. Even though tramadol is a centrally acting, synthetic opioid, primarily used for pain management, it is highly effective in the management of selected chronic cough cases. Furthermore, for that purpose it may be used in small doses, and it appears to not be particularly habit forming. It is a second-choice neurogenic cough medication.

**Transition phase (phase two), transition.** Phase after the induction (detox) reflux diet, characterized by modulation of the diet by trial and error with the goal of identifying trigger foods.

**Transnasal.** Literally, "through the nose," as in transnasal esophagoscopy. Usually an ultra-thin flexible endoscope is used for all types of transnasal diagnostics and procedures.

**Transnasal esophagoscopy (TNE).** Examination of the esophagus (and stomach), usually performed by an otolaryngologist without sedation. TNE is the best way to examine the esophagus in reflux patients; transnasal esophagoscopy is preferred because it is a safer, more accurate, and less expensive examination than EGD.

**Transnasal flexible laryngoscopy (TFL).** This is the state-of-the-art throat (larynx, voice box) examination method. After spraying the nose with a topical numbing agent, an ultra-thin flexible instrument (with a light and high-definition camera on the tip) is introduced through the nose and advanced into the upper throat. TFL is usually simultaneously performed with videostroboscopy, which allows closer examination of the vocal cords for growths, scarring, or vocal cord paresis. With subsequent video replay and still image capture, it allows the examiner to compute the reflux-finding score.

**Trigger foods**. Foods (or beverages) that cause reflux symptoms. A trigger food can be any food, and there is great individual variation from person to person. Banana, for example, pH 5.7, is generally considered to be a good-for-reflux fruit; unfortunately, banana is a trigger food for about 5 percent of people. The most common reflux trigger foods are chocolate, coffee, wine, nuts, onion, tomato, garlic, and pepper.

**Tuberculosis (TB)**. TB is still a significant cause of chronic cough in the Western world, and it should be ruled out by TB skin test and chest X-ray.

**UES**. *See upper esophageal sphincter.*

**Ultram**. *See tramadol.*

**Upper endoscopy**. Examination of the esophagus and stomach, sometimes the upper bowel as well. Endoscopy refers to examination performed by looking with a special instrument, an endoscope, from the inside, e.g., transnasal esophagoscopy.

**Upper-esophageal sphincter (UES)**. The valve at the upper end of the esophagus where it joins the pharynx (throat). Anatomically, the UES combines elements of both pharyngeal and esophageal muscles. The UES is responsible for preventing esophageal reflux from entering the airway. When it fails, airway reflux occurs. UES dysfunction, usually from airway reflux, is commonly responsible for globus (lump-in-the-throat sensation) symptoms.

**Upper respiratory infection (URI).** Generic name for a cold, the flu, or any infection that involves the nose and/or throat. URIs are believed to be responsible for post-viral vagal neuropathy.

**Vagal nerve.** See *vagus nerve.*

**Vagal nerve dysfunction.** Any abnormal function or problem that results from injury or damage to the vagus nerve; *dysfunction* literally means "bad function."

**Vagally mediated.** Caused by the vagus nerve; for example, neurogenic cough is vagally mediated.

**Vagus (vagal) nerve** (plural **vagi**). The vagus is the tenth cranial nerve; its origins are in the brainstem and it exits the skull to traverse the neck running in the carotid sheath with the carotid artery and the jugular vein. The vagi lie right under the lining membranes of the throat making them vulnerable to viral infections. The vagus is the primary nerve of the entire aerodigestive (airway and digestive) tract, including the vocal cords, the cough reflex, the esophagus and the esophageal sphincters, and the stomach. It even sends branches to the heart, ear, and colon. Post-viral vagal neuropathy may affect many different vagally mediated functions, especially cough.

**Videostroboscopy.** Videostroboscopy is performed during the laryngeal examination by transnasal flexible laryngoscopy (TFL). Videostroboscopy is really two functions: video recording of the examination for subsequent frame-by-frame play back and stroboscopy for ultra-slow-motion analysis of vocal cord movement. A floppy vocal cord on stroboscopy, for example, is characteristic of subtle vocal cord paresis as seen in post-viral vagal neuropathy.

**Viral inflammation**. Viral infections may affect infected tissues in such a way that inflammatory cells (white blood cells) are called into action. As a consequence, viral inflammation can lead to swelling, pain, and tissue damage. Viral inflammation may affect nerves as in Bell's palsy and post-viral vagal neuropathy.

**Vocal cord dysfunction (VCD)**. This is an outdated, non-specific diagnostic term that some physicians use to describe airway obstruction (breathing difficulties) at the laryngeal level. What makes this diagnosis is noise when breathing *in*, inspiratory stridor. VCD is a diagnosis generally used by clinicians incapable of laryngeal examination. Preferable is a specific diagnosis (after examination) such as reflux-related laryngospasm or paradoxical vocal cord movement.

**Vocal cord nerves**. The laryngeal (voice box) nerves that account for voice, cough, and airway protection during swallowing. The main vocal cord nerve is the recurrent laryngeal nerve; a second nerve, the superior laryngeal nerve, allows high-pitched voicing. All of these vocal cord (laryngeal) nerves are branches of the vagus.

**Vocal cord paralysis**. Complete immobility of a vocal cord leading to glottal closure symptoms; see also *vocal cord paresis* below.

**Vocal cord paresis**. Partial paralysis (weakness) leading to glottal closure symptoms such as vocal fatigue and effortful speaking, often due to post-viral vagal neuropathy.

**Voice disorders**. Any problem or disorder that leads to dysphonia (hoarseness). Voice disorders encompass nerve-muscle problems such as vocal cord paralysis and paresis, brain disorder problems such as Parkinsonism and spasmodic dysphonia, vocal cord growths such as nodules, polyps, and cancers, behavioral problems such as vocal abuse, misuse, or overuse syndromes and finally airway reflux.

**Wheezing**. Expiratory stridor, noisy breathing on exhalation, associated with asthma. Wheezing is associated with prolongation of the expiratory phase of respiration.

**Zenker's diverticulum**. An outpouching at the junction of the pharynx and upper esophagus that can trap undigested food and cause dysphagia (difficulty swallowing) and aspiration, usually seen in elderly patients. It is likely that Zenker's are caused by upper-esophageal-sphincter (value) dysfunction secondary to reflux. Fewer than half of these require surgical removal. Treatment with Botox injections is an alternative to surgery.

# INDEX

# ABOUT THE AUTHOR

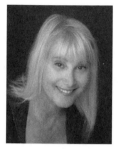

Dr. Jamie Koufman is one of America's leading laryngologists and has lectured widely, both nationally and internationally. With three decades of clinical and bench research focused on the diagnosis, treatment, cell biology, and epidemiology of reflux, Dr. Koufman is one of the world's authorities on reflux disease. She coined the terms *laryngopharyngeal reflux, silent reflux,* and *respiratory reflux.* She is a *New York Times* best-selling author for *Dropping Acid: The Reflux Diet Cookbook & Cure,* a book that offers refluxers good understanding of silent reflux and a natural cure. She is also the author of *Dr. Koufman's Acid Reflux Diet* and *Acid Reflux in Children.*

Dr. Koufman is the Founder and Director of the Voice Institute of New York, a comprehensive voice treatment center. She was a pioneer of laryngeal framework surgery, minimally-invasive laryngeal laser surgery, laryngeal electromyography, and transnasal esophagoscopy. Dr. Koufman is Professor of Clinical Otolaryngology at the New York Eye and Ear Infirmary of the Mt. Sinai Medical System.

Dr. Koufman has received the Honor Award and the Distinguished Service Awards of the American Academy of Otolaryngology—Head and Neck Surgery, the Broyles-Maloney Award of the American Broncho-Esophagological Association, and the Casselberry and Newcomb Awards of the American Laryngological Association. The latter is a lifetime achievement award for research and publications in Laryngology. She is a past president of the American Broncho-Esophagological Association and is currently the president of New York Laryngology Society. Dr. Koufman has been listed among the top doctors in America every year since 1994.